Total Joint Arthroplasty

Guest Editors

C. ALLYSON JONES, PT, PhD
LINDA C. LI, PT, PhD

CLINICS IN
GERIATRIC MEDICINE

www.geriatric.theclinics.com

August 2012 • Volume 28 • Number 3

SAUNDERS an imprint of ELSEVIER, Inc.

W.B. SAUNDERS COMPANY
A Division of Elsevier Inc.

1600 John F. Kennedy Blvd., Suite 1800. Philadelphia, Pennsylvania 19103-2899

http://www.theclinics.com

CLINICS IN GERIATRIC MEDICINE Volume 28, Number 3
August 2012 ISSN 0749-0690, ISBN-13: 978-1-4557-4933-1

Editor: Yonah Korngold

Clinics in Geriatric Medicine (ISSN 0749-0690) is published quarterly by Elsevier Inc., 360 Park Avenue South, New York, NY 10010-1710. Months of issue are February, May, August, and November. Business and Editorial Offices: 1600 John F. Kennedy Blvd., Suite 1800, Philadelphia, PA 191023-2899. Periodicals postage paid at New York, NY, and additional mailing offices. Subscription prices is $257.00 per year (US individuals), $448.00 per year (US institutions), $131.00 per year (US student/resident), $334.00 per year (Canadian individuals), $559.00 per year (Canadian institutions), $355.00 per year (foreign individuals) and $559.00 per year (foreign institutions). Foreign air speed delivery is included in all *Clinics* subscription prices. All prices are subject to change without notice. POSTMASTER: Send address changes to *Clinics in Geriatric Medicine,* Elsevier Health Sciences Division, Subscription Customer Service, 3251 Riverport Lane, Maryland Heights, MO 63043. Telephone: 1-800-654-2452 (U.S. and Canada); 314-447-8871 (outside U.S. and Canada). Fax: 314-447-8029. E-mail: journalscustomerservice-usa@elsevier.com (for print support) or journalsonlinesupport-usa@elsevier.com (for online support).

Reprints. For copies of 100 or more, of articles in this publication, please contact the Commercial Reprints Department, Elsevier Inc., 360 Park Avenue South, New York, New York 10010-1710. Tel.: (212) 633-3812; Fax: (212) 462-1935, email: reprints@elsevier.com.

Clinics in Geriatric Medicine is covered in *MEDLINE/PubMed (Index Medicus), EMBASE/Excerpta Medica, Current Contents/Clinical Medicine (CC/CM)*, and the *Cumulative Index to Nursing & Allied Health Literature.*

Printed and bound by CPI Group (UK) Ltd, Croydon, CR0 4YY
Transferred to Digital Print 2012

Contributors

GUEST EDITORS

C. ALLYSON JONES, PT, PhD
Associate Professor, Department of Physical Therapy, University of Alberta, Edmonton, Alberta, Canada

LINDA C. LI, PT, PhD
Associate Professor and Harold Robinson/Arthritis Society Chair in Arthritic Diseases, Department of Physical Therapy, University of British Columbia, Arthritis Research Centre of Canada, Richmond, British Columbia, Canada

AUTHORS

MEHRAN AGHAZADEH, MD
New England Baptist Hospital, Tufts University, Boston, Massachusetts

INGE VAN DEN AKKER-SCHEEK, PhD
Senior Researcher, Department of Orthopedics, University of Groningen, University Medical Center Groningen, Groningen, The Netherlands

ANDREW J. BARNETT, MRCS (Ed), FRCS (Trauma & Orth)
Knee Fellow, Exeter Knee Reconstruction Unit, Royal Devon and Exeter Hospital, Exeter, United Kingdom

MARISSA A. BLUM, MD, MS
Assistant Professor of Medicine, Division of Rheumatology, Temple University School of Medicine, Philadelphia, Pennsylvania

JAMES V. BONO, MD
Clinical Professor of Orthopedic Surgery, Tufts University, New England Baptist Hospital, Tufts University School of Medicine, Boston, Massachusetts

SJOERD K. BULSTRA, MD, PhD
Orthopedic Surgeon, Head, Department of Orthopedics, University of Groningen, University Medical Center Groningen, Groningen, The Netherlands

NATALIE J. COLLINS, PhD, PT
Postdoctoral Research Fellow, Department of Mechanical Engineering; Lecturer, Department of Physiotherapy, The University of Melbourne, Victoria, Australia

RAJIV GANDHI, MSc, MD, FRCSC
Assistant Professor, Division of Orthopaedics, Department of Surgery, Toronto Western Hospital, University Health Network, University of Toronto, Toronto, Ontario, Canada

SAID A. IBRAHIM, MD, MPH
Department of Medicine, Philadelphia VA Medical Center; Professor, Department of Medicine, The University of Pennsylvania School of Medicine, Philadelphia, Pennsylvania

C. ALLYSON JONES, PT, PhD
Associate Professor, Department of Physical Therapy, University of Alberta, Edmonton, Alberta, Canada

RICK L. LAU, MSc, MD, FRCSC
Clinical Fellow, Division of Orthopaedics, Department of Surgery, Toronto Western Hospital, University Health Network, University of Toronto, Toronto, Ontario, Canada

NIZAR MAHOMED, MD, ScD, FRCSC
Associate Professor and Head, Division of Orthopaedics, Department of Surgery, Toronto Western Hospital, University Health Network, University of Toronto, Toronto, Ontario, Canada

SAFIYYAH MAHOMED, BSc
Research Assistant, Division of Orthopaedics, Department of Surgery, Toronto Western Hospital, University Health Network, University of Toronto, Toronto, Ontario, Canada

ABDEL K. MEHIO, MD
Director, The Pain and Regional Anesthesia Program; Assistant Professor of Anesthesiology New England Baptist Hospital, Boston University School of Medicine, Boston, Massachusetts

SHERI POHAR, BScPharm, PhD
Canadian Agency for Drugs and Technologies in Health, Edmonton, Alberta, Canada

INGE H.F. REININGA, PhD
Senior Researcher, Department of Traumatology, University of Groningen, University Medical Center Groningen; Department of Orthopedics, Martini Hospital Groningen, Groningen, The Netherlands

CLAIRE E. ROBBINS, DPT
Research Assistant, Department of Orthopedic Surgery, New England Baptist Hospital, Tufts University, Boston, Massachusetts

EWA M. ROOS, PhD, PT
Professor, Research Unit for Musculoskeletal Function and Physiotherapy, Institute of Sports Science and Clinical Biomechanics, University of Southern Denmark, Odense M, Denmark

MARTIN STEVENS, PhD
Research Coordinator, Department of Orthopedics, University of Groningen, University Medical Center Groningen, Groningen, The Netherlands

CARL T. TALMO, MD
Associate Clinical Professor of Orthopedic Surgery, Tufts University, New England Baptist Hospital, Tufts University School of Medicine, Boston, Massachusetts

ANDREW D. TOMS, MSc, FRCS (Trauma & Orth), FRC (Ed)
Consultant Orthopaedic Surgeon, Exeter Knee Reconstruction Unit, Royal Devon and Exeter Hospital, Exeter, United Kingdom

ROBERT WAGENMAKERS, MD, PhD
Orthopedic Surgeon, Department of Orthopedics, Amphia Hospital Breda, Breda, The Netherlands

MARIE D. WESTBY, BSc (PT), PhD
Physical Therapy Teaching Supervisor, Mary Pack Arthritis Program; Clinical Associate Professor, Department of Physical Therapy, University of British Columbia, Vancouver, British Columbia, Canada

Contents

Patient satisfaction is an important outcome measurement in total knee arthroplasty/total hip arthroplasty surgery. Patient satisfaction can be evaluated from 2 perspectives, determinants of satisfaction and components of satisfaction. In total joint arthroplasty, improvements in satisfaction can be achieved by examining these perspectives. Patient satisfaction is one of the many PROMs (Patient Reported Outcome Measures) used in orthopedic surgery and is an integral part of the growing sentiment to evaluate surgery from the patient's perspective as well as from the surgeon's. The importance of measuring outcomes from the patient perspective is integral to today's patient centered models of care.

Total hip arthroplasty (THA) and total knee arthroplasty (TKA) are effective surgical interventions for relieving pain and improving physical function in patients with end-stage degenerative joint disease. Optimization of surgical outcomes requires selection of suitable patients, as well as postoperative evaluation utilizing appropriate patient-reported outcome measures. This article evaluates patient-reported outcomes frequently used for THA and TKA patients, including disease-specific (HOOS, HOOS-PS, KOOS, KOOS-PS, WOMAC), intervention-specific (Harris Hip Score, Oxford Hip Score, Oxford Knee Score), and generic instruments (EQ-5D, SF-12, SF-36), and provides a guide regarding their suitability for use in such patients based on their characteristics and psychometric properties.

This review examines recovery after total hip and knee arthroplasty. It aims to (1) provide an overview of the different types of disease-specific, generic, and utility outcome measures used to assess recovery after total hip and knee arthroplasty and (2) summarize reported changes in health-related quality of life after total joint arthroplasty.

Disease-specific measures reported large and important changes (assessed with minimally clinically important differences and effect size criteria), primarily for pain and function over short- and long-term recovery. Smaller but important changes were reported with generic and utility measures. Changes were largest in the pain and physical function domains.

The number of primary and revision total joint arthroplasty procedures is increasing exponentially with time. It is anticipated that there will be a huge expected demand for revision knee surgery over the next 2 decades. Awareness is needed by both general practitioner and physician for the signs of failure of these implants and when to refer to the surgeon. Unless the surgeon accurately identifies the mode of failure, successful treatment becomes very unlikely. In comparison with primary joint arthroplasty, complication rates after revision surgery are significantly increased, and outcome is less assured.

Total hip arthroplasty and total knee arthroplasty have proven to be effective surgical procedures for the treatment of hip and knee osteoarthritis. In recent decades, there have been considerable efforts to improve the component designs, modes of fixation, and surgical techniques. Minimally invasive techniques are examples of these developments. Minimally invasive total joint arthroplasty aims at decreasing the surgical incision and minimizing damage to the underlying soft tissue to accelerate postoperative recovery and an earlier return to normal function. The objective here is to report on these recent developments in minimally invasive total joint arthroplasty and their implication for the elderly patient.

Total knee replacement (TKR) and total hip replacement (THR) can provide pain relief and restoration of function in individuals with musculoskeletal impairment. The procedures are extremely successful and essentially unrivaled in the treatment of osteoarthritis pain. Demand is expected to increase. Because of these factors, a detailed understanding of perioperative issues in THR and TKR is important to practitioners. Issues include nonoperative measures and pharmacologic strategies. The discussion of pharmacology in joint replacement before, during, and after surgery includes multimodal management and agents such as acetaminophen, nonsteroidal antiinflammatory agents, injections of cortisone or visco-supplementation, and tramadol.

Total joint replacement (TJR) of the hip and knee is an effective procedure resulting in decreased pain and improved function in osteoarthritis patients. TJR is increasing at a significant rate, and increased awareness of potential complications following TJR is of paramount importance to all practitioners. The geriatric patient may be more susceptible to perioperative complications following TJR; therefore, careful preoperative planning, close perioperative monitoring, and the institution of appropriate preventative measures can minimize complications or dampen their impact. Complications to consider in the elderly patient following TJR include infection, thromboembolism, fracture, hip dislocation, and delirium, as well as cardiovascular complications.

Total joint arthroplasty surgeries are on the rise due to the aging population and the contribution of rising obesity rates to hip and knee osteoarthritis. With the growing demand, greater attention needs to be directed toward identifying cost-effective rehabilitation interventions to optimize outcomes in the long term. Patients' rehabilitation needs should be considered along a continuum with appropriate assessment and management of preoperative health and psychosocial issues and provision of exercise therapy postoperatively. The goal is to help patients adopt or resume physically active lifestyles, maintain their independence, and minimize reductions in functional capacity associated with normal aging.

Total hip (THA) and knee arthroplasty (TKA) are successful operative interventions, yet little is known about the physical activity behavior of patients after THA/TKA. For older adults, there are beneficial effects of regular physical activity after THA/TKA. The objective of this paper is to review the benefits of physical activity after THA/TKA, the potential negative consequences of physical activity on hip or knee prosthesis, the measurement of physical activity, physical activity behavior, and the current opinion of health care professionals regarding types of physical activities recommended for patients after THA/TKA.

Osteoarthritis is the most prevalent form of arthritis for which elective knee and hip joint replacement are effective treatment options in the management of end-stage disease. There are marked racial disparities in the utilization of joint arthroplasty. This article reviews the rationale for understanding this disparity, the evidence base that supports the disparity, and some known potential explanations, as well as additional data on racial disparities emerging in research on postarthroplasty outcomes and quality of care. The article concludes with a call for more research examining patient, provider and system-level factors that underlie these disparities.

CLINICS IN GERIATRIC MEDICINE

Preface

Total Joint Arthroplasty

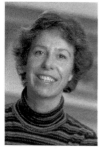 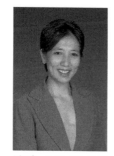

C. Allyson Jones, PT, PhD   Linda C. Li, PT, PhD
Guest Editors

Total knee arthroplasty and total hip arthroplasty are arguably the most cost-effective interventions for treating severe arthritis.[1] Approximately 95% of the procedures are received by patients with osteoarthritis.[2] With the population aging, demands for total joint arthroplasty will increase drastically. The advances in surgical techniques, as well as management before and after surgery, are truly remarkable. Our recent Medline search found over 1100 randomized controlled trials, involving patients undergoing total knee or hip arthroplasty, published in the past 20 years. Clinicians working with older patients have great interest in this topic, but it is indeed a daunting task to keep abreast with the large volume of new knowledge. Hence, it is exciting that *Clinics in Geriatric Medicine* dedicate this issue to total joint arthroplasty.

We have gathered an outstanding international group of authors to contribute to this issue. A decision was made to select topics that focus on patients rather than purely a clinical perspective of the condition or treatment. Topics also span the continuum of care for total joint arthroplasty. The first three articles synthesize the evidence of patient-centered outcomes after surgery. These include patient satisfaction of the procedures, physical function, and health-related quality of life. The next two articles focus on procedures that are particularly relevant to older patients, namely minimally invasive techniques and revision surgery. With continuing advances in prosthetic design and improvements in surgical and perioperative care, this issue provides practicing clinicians with recent evidence for effective management of patients with joint arthroplasty. We dedicate four articles to address advances in postarthroplasty management, including pharmaceutical interventions, complication management, rehabilitation, and return-to-activity interventions.

Clin Geriatr Med 28 (2012) xi–xii
http://dx.doi.org/10.1016/j.cger.2012.06.002
0749-0690/12/$ – see front matter © 2012 Elsevier Inc. All rights reserved.

geriatric.theclinics.com

This issue ends with a review on the disparity in access to surgical care. We end on this note with the intention to generate further interest and action to improve care especially for patients who are hard to reach, such as those living in rural and remote communities and the homeless population.

C. Allyson Jones, PT, PhD
Department of Physical Therapy
University of Alberta
2-50 Corbett Hall
Edmonton, AB, Canada T6G 2G4

Linda C. Li, PT, PhD
Department of Physical Therapy
University of British Columbia
Arthritis Research Centre of Canada
5591 No. 3 Road
Richmond, BC, Canada V6X 2C7

E-mail addresses:
cajones@ualberta.ca (C.A. Jones)
lli@arthritisresearch.ca (L.C. Li)

REFERENCES

1. Zhang W, Moskowitz RW, Nuki G, et al. OARSI recommendations for the management of hip and knee osteoarthritis, Part II: OARSI evidence-based, expert consensus guidelines. Osteoarthritis Cartilage 2008;16(2):137–62.
2. Quintana JM, Arostegui I, Escobar A, et al. Prevalence of knee and hip osteoarthritis and the appropriateness of joint replacement in an older population. Arch Intern Med 2008;168(14):1576–84.

Patient Satisfaction after Total Knee and Hip Arthroplasty

Rick L. Lau, MSc, MD, FRCSC[a], Rajiv Gandhi, MSc, MD, FRCSC[b],
Safiyyah Mahomed, BSc[c], Nizar Mahomed, MD, ScD, FRCSC[c],*

KEYWORDS

- Satisfaction • Knee arthroplasty • Hip arthroplasty • Patient-reported outcomes
- Dissatisfaction

KEY POINTS

- Patient satisfaction is an important outcome measurement in TKA/THA surgery.
- Patient satisfaction can be evaluated from 2 perspectives, determinants of satisfaction and components of satisfaction.
- Patient satisfaction is one of the many PROMs (Patient Reported Outcome Measures) used in orthopedic surgery and is an integral part of the growing sentiment to evaluate surgery from the patient's perspective as well as from the surgeon's.
- The importance of measuring outcomes from the patient perspective is integral to today's patient-centered models of care.

INTRODUCTION

In the developed world, arthritis is a leading cause of disability, and current estimates indicate that the total number of people with arthritis will double in the next 10 years.[1,2] Total hip arthroplasty (THA) and total knee arthroplasty (TKA) are 2 popular and effective surgical procedures to treat arthritis, with the total number of procedures expected to increase by more than 600% for TKA and by almost 200% for THA in the United States over the next 20 years.[3,4] The effectiveness of these procedures has been well established in the literature, and traditionally studies on THA and TKA have focused on clinically objective surgeon-reported endpoints, such as implant survivorship, range of motion, and radiographic results.[3]

The authors have nothing to disclose.
[a] Division of Orthopaedics, Department of Surgery, Toronto Western Hospital, University Health Network, University of Toronto, 399 Bathurst Street, EW 1-449, Toronto, ON M5T 2S8, Canada;
[b] Division of Orthopaedics, Department of Surgery, Toronto Western Hospital, University Health Network, University of Toronto, 399 Bathurst Street, EW 1-439, Toronto, ON M5T 2S8, Canada;
[c] Division of Orthopaedics, Department of Surgery, Toronto Western Hospital, University Health Network, University of Toronto, 399 Bathurst Street, EW 1-435, Toronto, ON M5T 2S8, Canada
* Corresponding author.
E-mail address: nizar.mahomed@uhn.on.ca

The trend of surgeon-reported outcomes, however, has come to change. With the effectiveness of medical care being increasingly measured both economically and clinically, patients' opinions have become increasingly important.[5] This development paralleled an increasing sociologic interest in the patient–doctor relationship and the demonstration of the importance of patients' opinions of their medical care.[5] This has led to the development of patient-reported outcome measures (PROMs), which are now a crucial aspect of evaluating health care outcomes and, more specifically, outcomes in THA and TKA.[6,7] In the United Kingdom, PROMs are also being introduced as a discriminating factor in health care funding and commissioning by hospitals.[7] Furthermore, it has been shown that patient- and physician-reported outcomes are not similar, with patient-reported outcomes often worse.[8] A meta-analysis has shown that physician and patient perceptions differ on many aspects of care, especially subjective quality-of-life domains, such as social and emotional well-being.[8] This has been seen in primary care settings as well as in orthopedics.[9,10]

All of the above have fueled the development and validation of PROMs in orthopedic surgery. There are several validated PROMs for measuring outcomes following THA and TKA, including, but not limited to, the generic 36-item Short Form Health survey (SF-36), 12-item Short Form Health survey (SF-12), the Western Ontario and McMaster University Osteoarthritis Index (WOMAC), the Oxford Hip Score (OHS), and the Oxford Knee Score. In keeping with this increased use of PROMs to measure outcome after THA and TKA, there is increasing interest in the measurement of patient satisfaction after these procedures.[7] Arguably, long-term satisfaction is the most important goal of surgery in patients with arthritis; thus, it is of paramount importance that it be measured and studied.[11] This review will examine patient satisfaction surrounding THA and TKA procedures as well as the factors that influence satisfaction and how to potentially improve on our current results.

THE CONCEPT OF PATIENT SATISFACTION

Ware and colleagues[12] have been credited with much of the theory behind the concept of patient satisfaction.[5] They made a distinction between objective satisfaction reports about providers and care (such as clinic waiting times) and satisfaction ratings—a patient's subjective evaluation of care.[12] This subjective evaluation of patient care or satisfaction reflected 3 variables: the personal preferences of the patient, the patient's expectations, and the technical aspects of the care received.[12] Building on this theory, Sitzia and Wood[5] stated that patient satisfaction is both a measure of the care received as well as a reflection of the patient. Accordingly, patient satisfaction can be examined from the viewpoint of determinants of satisfaction (patient variables such as age and expectations) and components of satisfaction (aspects of care received such as hospital environment and surgical techniques). Both the determinants of satisfaction and the components of satisfaction are helpful in providing a framework from which patient satisfaction can be examined as it relates to THA/TKA outcomes.

WHY IS PATIENT SATISFACTION IMPORTANT?

Measurements of patient satisfaction are important, as they accomplish several goals. The simplest of these goals is a description of health care from the patient's point of view, but taken further, studies of patient satisfaction reflect an evaluation of the health care process.[5] Indeed, some view patient satisfaction solely as a means to evaluate health care.[13] Donabedian[14] proposed that health care systems be evaluated in terms of structure, process, and outcome. *Structure* refers to the organization of the institution providing the care, including the environment within which the care is delivered; *process* refers to the professional activities surrounding the provision of care; and *outcome* refers to the change in a patient's health status secondary to the intervention.[14] To this end, patient satisfaction uniquely incorporates all of these aspects of care, making it a valuable metric in health care evaluation. In orthopedics and, more specifically, THA/TKA surgery, patient satisfaction provides a means of evaluating the many facets of care. Knowledge of the factors that affect satisfaction will allow for strategies to improve patient care in orthopedics.

HOW IS PATIENT SATISFACTION MEASURED?

Patient satisfaction surveys or questionnaires are a form of PROM and thus are subject to the same rigorous testing protocols inherent to all validated PROMs. More specifically, any measure of patient satisfaction must be tested and validated through psychometric analysis.[6] Psychometric analysis is the process of applying scientific methodology to the measurement of subjective outcomes or, as it pertains to this review, the validation of satisfaction questionnaires. It is usually composed of 3 components—validity, reliability, and responsiveness with validity and reliability being the minimum requirement for any PROM.[5]

Validity refers to how well the given test measures the question of interest. *Content validity* addresses whether a questionnaire has enough items and adequately covers the domain of interest.[6] Questionnaires with content validity cover the target behavior well and subsequently provide valid inferences.[6] Criterion validity is a comparison of the questionnaire with an existing, validated gold standard that is well accepted in the field.[15] Unfortunately, there is no widely accepted gold standard in assessing patient satisfaction after THA/TKA.

In the absence of a gold standard for comparison, one must assess validity using constructs. Construct validity may be obtained by comparing the test against another previously validated questionnaire or consensus statement.[6,16] Further means of obtaining construct validity involve the use of convergent and discriminant methods, whereby the results of the questionnaire correlate with other observable outcomes to which it should be related (convergent) and vice versa (discriminant).[6,16]

Reliability refers to the ability of a questionnaire to produce an outcome that remains unchanged when applied at different times, and no clinical change has occurred. *Test-retest reliability* refers to the variation in outcome measurements taken by a person under the same conditions at different time points. It measures reliability across time and can be measured using interclass coefficient values. Interrater reliability is an assessment of the degree to which different observers/testers give consistent estimates of the outcome being measured. This measures reliability of a test when administered by different people and can be measured by Cronbach's alpha (CA).[15]

Responsiveness refers to the ability of a questionnaire to detect change when applied at 2 different times when a change has, in fact, occurred. Responsiveness can be measured by calculating the standard effect size. Standard effect size is a measure of the change in the measured outcome from 1 interval to another divided by the standard deviation of the outcome at the initial interval.[17] Many PROMs in orthopedic surgery have demonstrated excellent responsiveness because of the large standard effect size associated with THA/TKA surgery.[18] This, however, has created problems as noted by Dunbar,[6] as subtle changes or variables in the intervention (such as using a different implant for THA/TKA) may be lost or masked by the large impact of THA/TKA intervention on PROMs.

In the past, patient satisfaction questionnaires have been notoriously inadequate when examined using psychometric principles. Sitzia and Wood[5] reviewed patient satisfaction studies and found that of 181 studies, only 6% of them utilized psychometric principles in the evaluation of the reliability and validity of the metric utilized to measure satisfaction. Of these 6 studies, none were specific to THA/TKA surgery or even to orthopedic surgery in general.

In 2011, Mahomed and coworkers[19] developed a patient satisfaction scale for use in THA/TKA surgery. The scale was tested using psychometric principles and found to have appropriate reliability as tested by CA scores (THA CA = 0.86 [12 weeks] and 0.91 [1 year], TKA CA = 0.91 [12 weeks] and 0.92 [1 year]). Construct validity was measured by comparing the satisfaction scale to SF-36 physical component score and WOMAC results.[20,21] In 2001, a single-item satisfaction questionnaire was tested by Dunbar[6] and Robertsson and colleagues.[11] It was found to demonstrate appropriate reliability and validity when tested on a large population in Sweden after TKA surgery. Reliability was measured with the use of Kappa coefficient testing (0.64 indicating good reliability).[6] Construct validity was measured with the use of WOMAC, SF-36, SF-12, Oxford Knee Score, and Nottingham Health Profile.[18,20-23] These 2 tests are to this author's knowledge the only patient satisfaction tests that have been demonstrated to have validity and reliability as tested on hip and knee arthroplasty patients.

SATISFACTION IN TKA

Results on satisfaction after TKA have generally been high, but there is a population of patients that are dissatisfied after surgery. Mahomed and coworkers[19] reported on 857 TKA patients and described an overall satisfaction score of 88% 1 year postoperatively. Similarly, Dunbar[6] and Robertsson and colleagues[11] reported on patient satisfaction from the Swedish Joint Arthroplasty Registry. They reported on 25,275 patients after TKA with a satisfaction rate of 81%. Both of these studies utilized a validated metric.

The above results compare well with those of other studies that have utilized nonvalidated questionnaires in the literature. Bourne and coworkers[24] reported an 81% satisfaction rate on 1375 patients after TKA, and Scott and colleagues[25] reported on 1290 TKAs with a satisfaction rate of 81.4%. Similarly, a study in 2011 reported a satisfaction rate of 89.8% in a study cohort of 264 patients.[26] Noble and coworkers[27] reported a 75% satisfaction rate in 253 patients. Anderson and colleagues[28] reported an 89% satisfaction rate in a cohort of patients over the age of 75. Gandhi and coworkers[29] reported a satisfaction rate at the time of surgery of 92.2%, but this included results for both hip and knee arthroplasty.

There are also studies that measure patient satisfaction after TKA, utilizing a visual analog scale (VAS). Bullens and coworkers[10] reported a VAS of 80 points on a 100-point scale, (100 = best score) in 128 patients. Similarly, Husted and colleagues[30] reported a mean overall satisfaction of 9.3 on a 10-point scale (10 = best score) in 342 patients. Unfortunately, VAS does not identify which patients are satisfied and which are not, making it somewhat difficult to interpret. Some investigators have suggested that because satisfaction is uniformly high, it is more important to focus on the unsatisfied or dissatisfied group.[31-33] In the dissatisfied group lies the opportunity for insight and subsequent changes to decrease the proportion of those who are dissatisfied.[31-33] Patient satisfaction data derived from VAS do not allow for identification of the dissatisfied patient, as there is no defined threshold VAS for which

Table 1 Determinants of satisfaction in TKA	
Variable	Effect on Satisfaction
Age	±ve
Gender	No effect
Psychiatric comorbidity	−ve
Patient expectation	−ve (expectation not met) +ve (high expectation of pain relief)
Medical comorbidity	−ve (other arthritic joints, back pain)
Diagnosis	+ve (rheumatoid arthritis)
Severity of disease	−ve (low preoperative WOMAC) −ve (high pain at rest) +ve (severe radiographic evidence of OA)

Abbreviations: OA, osteoarthritis; −ve, negative effect on satisfaction; +ve, positive effect on satisfaction; ±ve, unclear effect on satisfaction.

a patient can be labeled dissatisfied. This highlights the difficulty in understanding patient satisfaction data derived from VAS scores and patient satisfaction data in general.

DETERMINANTS OF SATISFACTION IN TKA

The determinants of satisfaction have been described by Sitzia and Wood[5] as all of the patient-related factors that affect the patients' subjective experience of the proposed treatment. There have been many postulated patient factors ranging from simple factors, such as age, to more complex factors, such as patient expectation, that may affect patient satisfaction (**Table 1**).

Patient Age

Patient age has long been postulated to affect satisfaction with TKA. Bourne and colleagues[24] reported that advancing patient age was a predictor of patient dissatisfaction. In contrast, Merle-Vincent and colleagues[26] found that age greater than 70 was a positive predictor of patient satisfaction. Both Gandhi and coworkers[25] and Scott and coworkers[29] found no difference with age, and, still more confusing, Noble and colleagues[27] reported that young age was associated with higher satisfaction and age 60 to 75 was associated with lower satisfaction. It is likely that physiologic age is more important than chronologic age, with fitter, more active older patients behaving more like younger patients, and vice versa.[27] Clearly, it is not well understood how age affects satisfaction.

Patient Gender

Gender does not appear to affect satisfaction in TKA. This has been shown in multiple reports and appears to be well elucidated.[24–27,29]

Patient Expectations

Patients' expectations are also emerging as a very important determinant of patient satisfaction. Mahomed and colleagues[2] found that patients who had low expectation of complications preoperatively had higher levels of satisfaction, and patients who expected complete pain relief had higher levels of pain relief and function postoperatively. Bourne and coworkers[24] found that the largest contributing factor to patient dissatisfaction was not meeting patients' expectations, with an odds ratio of more than 10. Furthermore, Scott and colleagues[25] found patient satisfaction to correlate well with meeting patients' expectations. It is clear that patients' expectations have a large impact on patient satisfaction, and management of patients' expectations may help surgeons decrease the proportion of dissatisfied patients.

Psychiatric Comorbidity

Mental health also appears to play a role in satisfaction. Scott and coworkers[25] and Brander and coworkers[34] both found an association between poor mental health and dissatisfaction with TKA. In 2008, Gandhi and colleagues[29] identified learned helplessness as a significant negative predictor of WOMAC change after total joint arthroplasty. Similarly, it has also been found that patients who tend to catastrophize their pain have higher postsurgical pain after TKA and poorer postsurgical function.[35] Depression has also been identified as a negative predictor of function as well as postoperative pain relief.[35,36] In 2009, Gandhi and colleagues[37] found that patients reporting higher levels of mental health dysfunction had a statistically higher chance of being dissatisfied after total joint arthroplasty.

Medical Comorbidity

Medical comorbidities have an unclear impact on patient satisfaction. Gandhi and coworkers[38] reported no significant impact of medical comorbidities on patient satisfaction using the Charlson index. Similarly, Bourne and colleagues[24] reported that there was no effect of medical comorbidities as measured by American Society of Anesthesiologists class. In contrast, Scott and coworkers[25] found that there was a small but significant increase in dissatisfaction in patients with a higher number of medical comorbidities (1.1 v 1.4). A closer examination of the comorbidities that were tested found a very high correlation between back pain, depression, and other painful joints and patient dissatisfaction.[25] This is not a surprising result, as it would make sense that musculoskeletal comorbidities may alter a patient's ability to rehabilitate completely after TKA and obtain full benefit from TKA.[25] Separation of medical comorbidities from musculoskeletal comorbidities may help clarify the role of each in patient satisfaction.

Diagnosis Leading to TKA

The patient's diagnosis leading to TKA appears to affect patient satisfaction. In 2000, Robertsson and colleagues[11] reported a higher satisfaction rate in patients with rheumatoid arthritis compared with patients with a preoperative diagnosis of osteoarthritis, osteonecrosis, or posttraumatic arthritis. They postulated that patients with rheumatoid arthritis may be more satisfied with relief of pain, whereas patients with other diagnoses may expect a return to their premorbid function.[11] Similarly, Bullens and colleagues[10] suggested that patients with rheumatoid arthritis had lower expectations and subsequently met their expectations more readily after surgery, leading to higher satisfaction rates.

Severity of Arthropathy

The severity of symptoms before TKA appears to impact patient satisfaction. Bourne and colleagues[24] found that patients with high levels of pain at rest, sitting, or lying were more likely to be dissatisfied after surgery. Similarly, they reported that patients

Table 2	
Components of satisfaction in TKA	
Variable	Effect on Satisfaction
Anesthetic	+ve (local anesthetic infiltration)
Surgical incision	±ve
Type of components	±ve
Computer assisted	No effect
Postoperative rehabilitation	±ve
Postoperative complications	−ve (postoperative complications requiring admission to hospital)

Abbreviations: +ve, positive effect on satisfaction; ±ve, unclear effect on satisfaction.

with poor WOMAC scores for pain and function preoperatively were more likely to be dissatisfied,[24] a result echoed by Kim and coworkers.[39] These results are in agreement with studies that have demonstrated poor preoperative WOMAC scores to be predictive of poor postoperative WOMAC scores.[40–42] In contrast, Gandhi and colleagues[38] found no significant effect of preoperative WOMAC scores on patient satisfaction but did find a significant correlation between poor preoperative SF-36 mental health scores and dissatisfaction. Merle-Vincent and coworkers[26] found that patients with more severe radiographic findings were more likely to be satisfied postoperatively. Dissatisfied patients were more likely to have less radiographic joint space narrowing than their satisfied counterparts.[26]

Unresolved Pain

Two large studies have examined patients who were not satisfied with TKA and found that unresolved pain was a significant factor. Scott and colleagues[25] found that a lack of improvement in pain in the operated knee was the most significant factor in predicting dissatisfaction with TKA. Similarly, Dunbar[6] reported on patient satisfaction after TKA in a large cohort of Swedish patients. The satisfaction of patients correlated well with pain relief and improved function.

COMPONENTS OF SATISFACTION IN TKA

The components of satisfaction are all of the processes and technical aspects of TKA that can affect patient satisfaction. This ranges from the type of anesthetic administered, the technical aspects of the surgery itself, and all of the health care processes such as rehabilitation programs (**Table 2**).

Anesthetic Factors

There are many aspects of anesthesia that can be evaluated in terms of patient satisfaction in TKA; however, there is a paucity of evidence. There is some evidence published comparing local infiltration anesthesia versus epidural anesthesia for postoperative pain. Thorsell and colleagues[43] reported higher rates of satisfaction with local anesthetic versus continuous epidural anesthesia, with 77% being very satisfied after local anesthesia versus 40% for epidural anesthesia for postoperative analgesia. Similarly, Busch and colleagues[44] found that local infiltration anesthetic improved patient satisfaction compared with patient-controlled analgesia.

Surgical Incision

Minimally invasive (MIS) TKA has been studied recently in the orthopedic literature as a potential means to improve patient outcomes.[39] A recent meta-analysis of the clinical and radiographic outcomes of conventional versus MIS techniques was performed by Smith and coworkers.[45] The analysis showed no difference in clinical or radiologic outcomes after MIS versus conventional techniques; however, patient satisfaction specifically was not examined in the analysis and remains largely unknown. Recently, Hernandez-Vaquero and colleagues[46] published data on MIS versus conventional incision TKA and patient satisfaction. They found no difference utilizing a VAS measurement tool for patient satisfaction. The VAS score for the MIS group was 8.3 (standard deviation [SD] 1.9) versus 8.2 (SD 1.3) in the traditional incision group.[46] This result is difficult to interpret because of the nature of VAS data as discussed earlier.

Type of Components

There are a variety of component designs, and several have been examined to see if there is an effect on patient satisfaction. Studies examining cemented versus uncemented,[47] posterior cruciate retaining versus posterior stabilized,[39,48] total versus unicompartmental knee arthroplasty,[11] patellar resurfaced versus nonresurfaced TKA,[49–52] all polyethylene tibia component versus metal backed tibia component TKA,[53] and oxidized zirconium versus cobalt chromium TKA[54] have all been performed and shown to have no significant impact on patient satisfaction. All of these studies highlight the potential difficulty in using PROMs to measure outcome after TKA, as the large standard effect size associated with TKA can mask any subtle impact that these factors may have on patient satisfaction.

Computer-Assisted TKA

As with MIS TKA, computer navigation has been investigated extensively as it relates to TKA surgery. Spencer and colleagues[55] found no statistically significant difference in patient satisfaction comparing computer-navigated TKA and conventional TKA 2 years after surgery. Similarly, Harvie and colleagues[56] reported no difference in patient satisfaction comparing computer-navigated TKA versus conventional TKA at a period of 5 years after surgery. It would appear that computer navigation does not have an effect on patient satisfaction.[56]

Postoperative Rehabilitation

In 2008, Mahomed and coworkers[57] found no significant difference in patient satisfaction when comparing inpatient rehabilitation with home-based rehabilitation after TKA. This result is further supported by the use of telemedicine in providing remote physiotherapy to patients after TKA. Russell and coworkers[58] reported high patient satisfaction when this form of rehabilitation was provided to patients in rural areas.

Postoperative Complications

Postoperative complications can have an impact on patient satisfaction. Bourne and coworkers[24] reported an odds ratio of 1.9 when examining the effect of a postoperative complication on dissatisfaction. Unfortunately, the various complications encountered were not identified. Further study of different postoperative complications may help identify which factors are particularly damaging to patient satisfaction and focus attention on improving outcomes.

SATISFACTION IN THA

Results of satisfaction after THA have universally been high, and THA is one of the most successful surgical procedures in the world. Hip arthroplasty satisfaction has

Table 3
Determinants of satisfaction in THA

Variable	Effect on Satisfaction
Age	±ve
Gender	±ve
Psychiatric comorbidity	±ve
Patient expectation	−ve (expectation not met) +ve (high expectation of pain relief)
Medical comorbidity	−ve (other arthritic joints, back pain)
Diagnosis	+ve (rheumatoid arthritis) −ve (hip dysplasia)
Severity of disease	No effect

Abbreviations: −ve, negative effect on satisfaction; +ve, positive effect on satisfaction; ±ve, unclear effect on satisfaction.

been reported from several studies, with most reports showing satisfaction around or above 90%.[7,24,59,60] Two studies have examined the difference between THA and TKA satisfaction, Bourne and coworkers[61] reported a THA satisfaction rate of 89% compared with that of TKA at 81% and Mahomed and colleagues[19] reported a THA satisfaction of 96.6% 1 year postoperatively for THA compared with 88% for TKA. These results are echoed by studies that have shown improved WOMAC function scores after THA compared with TKA.[41,62]

DETERMINANTS OF SATISFACTION IN THA

As with TKA, there are many postulated factors that may affect satisfaction. These are summarized in **Table 3**.

Age

The issue of age as a determinant of satisfaction has been examined for many years. Mancuso and colleagues[60] examined THA satisfaction and found no relationship between satisfied patients and age. Similarly, Anakwe and colleagues[7] found no difference in satisfaction rate when examining age. In contrast, Clement and coworkers[63] in 2011 found that patients older than 80 were more satisfied with THA compared with patients age 65 to 79, using a 6-point scale. Age remains to be an unclear determinant of satisfaction, likely for similar reasons as for TKA.

Gender

Similar to TKA surgery, there are several studies that have found gender does not appear to affect the rate of satisfaction in THA surgery.[7,29,64] However, Rolfson and colleagues[65] found that women had significantly lower health-related quality-of-life scores and satisfaction after THA. Their result is difficult to interpret, as they measured satisfaction using a VAS score out of 100 (100 = lowest satisfaction). Using this metric, men scored 15 and women 19. Although this may be statistically significant, it is unclear if a score of 19 means that patients are more likely to be unsatisfied with their surgery.

Patient Expectations

Patient expectations, as shown in TKA surgery, play an important role in patient satisfaction. Meeting patient expectations in THA surgery has been shown to correlate strongly with patient satisfaction.[7,60] Interestingly, higher patient expectations have been found to correlate well with improved pain relief postoperatively as well as function after joint arthroplasty.[3,38] Intuitively, managing patient expectations will help patients more consistently meet their expectations with the hope of higher levels of satisfaction.

Psychiatric Comorbidity

The impact of psychiatric illness or poor mental health on satisfaction after THA is unclear. Anakwe and colleagues[7] found that there was a correlation between poor mental component score on the SF-12 and a history of depression and dissatisfaction after THA when they analyzed their data using univariate analysis, but this finding was not significant after a multivariate analysis. In contrast, Gandhi and colleagues[29] found that there was a significant impact of mental health on patient satisfaction as measured by the mental component score of the SF-36. This study, however, involved both TKA and THA, making it difficult to interpret. Rolfson and colleagues found that patients with anxiety/depression scored significantly worse on VAS satisfaction score after THA,[65] especially if they remained anxious or depressed 1 year after surgery.[59] The effect of psychiatric comorbidity seems less clear in THA surgery compared with TKA surgery, but there does appear to be a general trend for psychiatric comorbidity having a negative impact on THA satisfaction. One potential reason the impact of psychiatric comorbidity on THA satisfaction is inconsistent may be the uniformly higher levels of satisfaction in this group than in the TKA group.[19] It is also possible that a more subtle relationship exists in the THA group as opposed to the TKA group, where results more consistently show a statistically significant impact. Further studies in the effect of psychiatric comorbidity on THA satisfaction are needed to understand this relationship.

Medical Comorbidity

The effect of medical comorbidities on THA satisfaction is similar to that for TKA. Anakwe and colleagues[7] found that symptomatic arthritis in another joint was associated with a significant increase in being dissatisfied after THA. Hossain and coworkers[66] reported no significant impact of medical comorbidity on THA satisfaction and Bourne and colleagues[61] echoed this result as well in their report. Rolfson and colleagues[59,65] found that comorbidity did affect postoperative satisfaction as measured using the Charnley comorbidity classification. It appears that musculoskeletal comorbidity such as back pain and other arthritic joints have a negative impact on satisfaction after THA. This concurs with the evidence found in TKA surgery.

Diagnosis Leading to THA

Diagnosis may play a role in satisfaction after THA. Rolfson and coworkers[59] found inflammatory arthritis to respond well to THA and for patients with inflammatory arthritis to have higher satisfaction than those with other diagnoses. Patients with a diagnosis of hip dysplasia were found to be significantly less satisfied.[67] Mancuso and colleagues[60] found no difference when examining diagnosis and satisfaction.

Severity of Arthropathy

In contrast to TKA, severity of symptoms has been found not to correlate with satisfaction in patients undergoing THA. Anakwe and coworkers[7] found that patients' preoperative SF-12 and OHS scores did not affect satisfaction. Arden and colleagues[64] found no association between baseline OHS and patient satisfaction.

Table 4	
Components of satisfaction in THA	
Variable	**Effect on Satisfaction**
Anesthetic	±ve
Surgical incision	±ve
Surgical approach	No effect
Implant fixation	±ve
Postoperative rehabilitation	+ve (aggressive postoperative rehabilitation)
	+ve (preoperative education on postoperative rehabilitation)
Postoperative complications	±ve

Abbreviations: +ve, positive effect on satisfaction; ±ve, unclear effect on satisfaction.

Similarly, Rolfson and colleagues[59] found that preoperative function and radiographic appearance were not associated with patient satisfaction. Furthermore, Gandhi and coworkers[29] found that preoperative function as measured by WOMAC scores did not affect patient satisfaction when examining THA and TKA.

COMPONENTS OF SATISFACTION IN THA

As for TKA, there are many "components of satisfaction" that can potentially affect patient satisfaction after THA. These are summarized in **Table 4**.

Anesthetic Factors

The use of spinal anesthetic in THA surgery was reported more than 30 years ago, with reported benefits of reduction in blood loss, deep venous thrombosis, and pulmonary embolism as outlined by a recent meta-analysis.[68] Unfortunately, it is still unclear as to whether there is a significant impact on patient satisfaction after THA. There have been many reports illustrating various postoperative analgesia regimens with some relevance to patient satisfaction. Busch and colleagues[69] reported on the use of local injection with morphine, ropivacaine, ketorolac, and epinephrine. This regimen was previously reported by the group to work well at reducing pain and improving satisfaction in TKA surgery in 2006.[44] They found a significant decrease in morphine use as well as pain postoperatively; however, there was no significant impact on patient satisfaction.[69] In 2004, Gurlit and colleagues[70] reported on improved patient satisfaction with continuous spinal analgesia versus continuous epidural analgesia. Furthermore, continuous epidural analgesia was found to improve patient satisfaction when comparing continuous epidural with patient-controlled analgesia.[71]

Unfortunately, the number of different medications used, the different anesthetic techniques performed (epidural/intradural/local/regional), and timing of patient evaluation (some measured satisfaction immediately after surgery, some upon discharge), make comparisons of different or even the same type of anesthetic difficult when examining patient satisfaction in THA.

Surgical Approach

Traditionally, there are 2 main approaches to the hip for THA surgery: posterior and direct lateral approaches.[45] Anakwe and coworkers[7] found no significant difference in satisfaction rates between patients operated via a posterior or lateral approach.

Surgical Incision

MIS THA has been a controversial topic in the orthopedic literature. Proponents exclaim lower postoperative pain, faster recovery of function, less muscle dissection and trauma, and similar complication rates to conventional THA.[45,71–73] Detractors exclaim higher risk of complications, muscle damage caused by retractor pressure and placement, and component malposition associated with MIS techniques.[45,71–73] Patient satisfaction is unclear as well, and to date no definitive answer has been established.

Implant Fixation

There are 2 main fixation techniques in THA surgery, cemented techniques and uncemented techniques, which apply to both the acetabular and femoral component. There are also hybrid techniques with cemented femoral stems and uncemented acetabular cups and vice versa. The majority of studies in the past have examined these techniques from the surgeon's perspective, often with survivorship as the main outcome. There is 1 study that demonstrated hybrid fixation techniques to have a higher satisfaction rate than uncemented techniques.[60] Unfortunately, authors do not elaborate on what hybrid technique was used (ie, cemented femur/uncemented cup or uncemented femur/cemented cup). Uncemented fixation of femoral components has been associated with thigh pain,[74] a potential explanation for the difference in satisfaction between the uncemented group and the hybrid group. Further study in this area would be of benefit in understanding its role in patient satisfaction after THA.

Postoperative Rehabilitation

In 2007, Pour and colleagues[75] found that patients involved in an accelerated rehabilitation program performed better postoperatively in terms of length of stay, patient satisfaction, and walking ability when compared with a standard protocol. The accelerated protocol included family education, patient preconditioning, preemptive analgesia with celecoxib, and an aggressive preoperative and postoperative physiotherapy regimen.[75] Interestingly, preoperative advice and education in the form of a "hip class" and information booklet have also been shown to improve patient satisfaction in THA.[76]

Postoperative Complications

In contrast with TKA, the presence of major perioperative complications did not appear to have a significant impact on patient satisfaction. Several studies have found no effect of complications on patient satisfaction.[7,60,66] Unfortunately, all of these studies do not list the various types of complications, and Anakwe and colleagues[7] admitted that there was a very low complication rate in their study, potentially leading to type 2 error. Interestingly, Iversen and coworkers[77] reported on perceived leg length discrepancy, a well known postoperative complication after THA. They found no correlation between perceived leg length discrepancy and patient satisfaction.[77]

Despite these studies, it would intuitively make sense that postoperative complications be associated with patient dissatisfaction after THA. It is difficult to know if this is a result of the large standard effect size associated with THA surgery masking more subtle variables, such as perceived leg length discrepancy. Further study in this area to determine its role in patient satisfaction is needed.

IMPROVING PATIENT SATISFACTION

Improving TKA/THA patient satisfaction is a difficult task, given the generally high satisfaction rates associated with each procedure. Still, there is a definable population of unsatisfied patients whose result may be influenced by altering some of the variables that affect patient satisfaction as it pertains to total joint replacement surgery.

For TKA patients, mental health has been found to affect patient satisfaction. Efforts to improve patient mental health preoperatively could represent an opportunity to influence patient satisfaction postoperatively. Meeting patient expectations has also been identified as an important predictor of patient satisfaction in both TKA and THA. A fine balance between keeping patient expectations high, as identified by Mahomed and coworkers,[2] and meeting patient expectations as identified by Bourne and colleagues,[24] is needed because both have been associated with higher patient satisfaction. Interestingly, a recent study by Mancuso and colleagues[78] in 2008 found an ability to alter expectations in TKA and THA using a preoperative education program. Preoperative education programs, centered on modifying patient expectations, may provide a mechanism to improve the rate of meeting patient expectations and, in turn, improve patient satisfaction.

Managing musculoskeletal comorbidities may also enhance patient satisfaction in TKA and THA. Prompt treatment of concomitant multiple joint arthritis may improve satisfaction after TKA and THA.

Surgical factors such as type of incision, surgical approach, type of implants, and surgical techniques have an unclear effect on patient satisfaction, and further research is required before any firm conclusions can be made. The same can be said of anesthetic factors; however, techniques that allow for improved postoperative pain control without impairing postoperative rehabilitation show promise for improving patient satisfaction.

Aggressive postoperative rehabilitation and education of patients with regard to expectations from physiotherapists and other allied health services during their postoperative recovery may provide additional means of improving patient satisfaction.

SUMMARY

Patient satisfaction is an important outcome measurement in TKA/THA surgery. Patient satisfaction can be evaluated from 2 perspectives, determinants of satisfaction and components of satisfaction.[5] In total joint arthroplasty, improvements in satisfaction can be achieved by examining these perspectives. Patient satisfaction is one of the many PROMs used in orthopedic surgery and is an integral part of the growing sentiment to evaluate surgery from the patient's perspective as well as from the surgeon's. The importance of measuring outcomes from the patient perspective is integral to today's patient-centered models of care.

REFERENCES

1. Alviar MJ, Olver J, Brand C, et al. Do patient-reported outcome measures in hip and knee arthroplasty rehabilitation have robust measurement attributes? A systematic review. J Rehabil Med 2011;43(7):572–83.
2. Mahomed NN, Liang MH, Cook EF, et al. The importance of patient expectations in predicting functional outcomes after total joint arthroplasty. J Rheumatol 2002;29(6): 1273–79.

3. Wylde V, Blom AW, Whitehouse SL, et al. Patient-reported outcomes after total hip and knee arthroplasty: comparison of midterm results. J Arthroplasty 2009;24(2): 210–16.

4. Kurtz S, Ong K, Lau E, et al. Projections of primary and revision hip and knee arthroplasty in the United States from 2005 to 2030. J Bone Joint Surg Am 2007; 89(4):780–5.

5. Sitzia J, Wood N. Patient satisfaction: a review of issues and concepts. Soc Sci Med 1997;45(12):1829–43.

6. Dunbar MJ. Subjective outcomes after knee arthroplasty. Acta Orthop Scand Suppl 2001;72(301):1–63.

7. Anakwe RE, Jenkins PJ, Moran M. Predicting dissatisfaction after total hip arthroplasty: a study of 850 patients. J Arthroplasty 2011;26(2):209–13.

8. Janse AJ, Gemke RJBJ, Uiterwaal CSPM, et al. Quality of life: patients and doctors don't always agree: a meta-analysis. J Clin Epidemiol 2004;57(7):653–61.

9. Mäntyselkä P, Kumpusalo E, Ahonen R, et al. Patients "versus general practitioners" assessments of pain intensity in primary care patients with non-cancer pain. Br J Gen Pract 2001;51(473):995–7.

10. Bullens PH, van Loon CJ, de Waal Malefijt MC, et al. Patient satisfaction after total knee arthroplasty: a comparison between subjective and objective outcome assessments. J Arthroplasty 2001;16(6):740–7.

11. Robertsson O, Dunbar M, Pehrsson T, et al. Patient satisfaction after knee arthroplasty: a report on 27,372 knees operated on between 1981 and 1995 in Sweden. Acta Orthop Scand 2000;71(3):262–7.

12. Ware JE, Snyder MK, Wright WR, et al. Defining and measuring patient satisfaction with medical care. Eval Program Plann 1983;6(3–4):247–63.

13. Bond S, Thomas LH. Measuring patients' satisfaction with nursing care. J Adv Nurs 1992;17(1):52–63.

14. Donabedian A. Evaluating the quality of medical care. 1966;2005:691–729.

15. Bland J, Altman D. Statistics notes: cronbach's alpha. BMJ 1997;314(22):572.

16. Sitzia J. How valid and reliable are patient satisfaction data? An analysis of 195 studies. Int J Qual Health Care 1999;11(4):319–28.

17. Wright JG, Young NL. A comparison of different indices of responsiveness. J Clin Epidemiol 1997;50(3):239–46.

18. Dawson J, Fitzpatrick R, Murray D, et al. Questionnaire on the perceptions of patients about total knee replacement. J Bone Joint Surg Br 1998;80(1):63–9.

19. Mahomed N, Gandhi R, Daltroy L, et al. The self-administered patient satisfaction scale for primary hip and knee arthroplasty. Arthritis 2011.

20. Bellamy N, Buchanan WW, Goldsmith CH, et al. Validation study of WOMAC: a health status instrument for measuring clinically important patient relevant outcomes to antirheumatic drug therapy in patients with osteoarthritis of the hip or knee. J Rheumatol 1988;15(12):1833–40.

21. McHorney CA, Ware JE, Raczek AE. The MOS 36-Item Short-Form Health Survey (SF-36): II. Psychometric and clinical tests of validity in measuring physical and mental health constructs. Medical Care 1993;31(3):247–63.

22. Hunt SM, McKenna SP, McEwen J, et al. A quantitative approach to perceived health status: a validation study. J Epidemiol Community Health 1980;34(4):281–6.

23. Ware J, Kosinski M, Keller SD. A 12-Item Short-Form Health Survey: construction of scales and preliminary tests of reliability and validity. Medical Care 1996;34(3): 220–33.

24. Bourne RB, Chesworth BM, Davis AM, et al. Patient Satisfaction after Total Knee Arthroplasty: Who is Satisfied and Who is Not? Clin Orthop Relat Res 2010;468(1): 57–63.
25. Scott CEH, Howie CR, MacDonald D, et al. Predicting dissatisfaction following total knee replacement: a prospective study of 1217 patients. J Bone Joint Surg Br 2010;92(9):1253–8.
26. Merle-Vincent F, Couris CM, Schott A-M, et al. Factors predicting patient satisfaction 2 years after total knee arthroplasty for osteoarthritis. Joint Bone Spine 2011;78(4): 383–6.
27. Noble PC, Conditt MA, Cook KF, et al. The John Insall Award: patient expectations affect satisfaction with total knee arthroplasty. Clin Orthop Relat Res 2006;452: 35–43.
28. Anderson JG, Wixson RL, Tsai D, et al. Functional outcome and patient satisfaction in total knee patients over the age of 75. J Arthroplasty 1996;11(7):831–40.
29. Gandhi R, Davey JR, Mahomed NN. Predicting patient dissatisfaction following joint replacement surgery. J Rheumatol 2008;35(12):2415–18.
30. Husted H, Holm G, Jacobsen S. Predictors of length of stay and patient satisfaction after hip and knee replacement surgery: fast-track experience in 712 patients. Acta Orthop 2008;79(2):168–73.
31. Fox JG, Storms DM. A different approach to sociodemographic predictors of satisfaction with health care. Soc Sci Med A 1981;15(5):557–64.
32. Carr-Hill RA. The measurement of patient satisfaction. J Public Health Med 1992; 14(3):236–49.
33. Williams B. Patient satisfaction: a valid concept? Soc Sci Med 1994;38(4):509–16.
34. Brander V, Gondek S, Martin E, et al. Pain and depression influence outcome 5 years after knee replacement surgery. Clin Orthop Relat Res 2007;464:21–6.
35. Sullivan M, Tanzer M, Stanish W, et al. Psychological determinants of problematic outcomes following Total Knee Arthroplasty. Pain 2009;143(1–2):123–29.
36. Sullivan M, Tanzer M, Reardon G, et al. The role of presurgical expectancies in predicting pain and function one year following total knee arthroplasty. Pain 2011; 152(10):2287–93.
37. Gandhi R, Razak F, Tso P, et al. Greater perceived helplessness in osteoarthritis predicts outcome of joint replacement surgery. J Rheumatol 2009;36(7):1507–11.
38. Gandhi R, Davey JR, Mahomed N. Patient expectations predict greater pain relief with joint arthroplasty. J Arthroplasty 2009;24(5):716–21.
39. Kim TK, Chang CB, Kang YG, et al. Causes and predictors of patient's dissatisfaction after uncomplicated total knee arthroplasty. J Arthroplasty 2009;24(2):263–71.
40. Lingard EA, Katz JN, Wright EA, et al, Kinemax Outcomes Group. Predicting the outcome of total knee arthroplasty. J Bone Joint Surg Am 2004;86-A(10):2179–86.
41. Fortin PR, Clarke AE, Joseph L, et al. Outcomes of total hip and knee replacement: preoperative functional status predicts outcomes at six months after surgery. Arthritis Rheum 1999;42(8):1722–8.
42. Fortin PR, Penrod JR, Clarke AE, et al. Timing of total joint replacement affects clinical outcomes among patients with osteoarthritis of the hip or knee. Arthritis Rheum 2002;46(12):3327–30.
43. Thorsell M, Holst P, Hyldahl HC, et al. Pain control after total knee arthroplasty: a prospective study comparing local infiltration anesthesia and epidural anesthesia. Orthopedics 2010;33(2):75–80.
44. Busch CA, Shore BJ, Bhandari R, et al. Efficacy of periarticular multimodal drug injection in total knee arthroplasty. A randomized trial. J Bone Joint Surg Am 2006;88(5):959–63.

45. Smith TO, Blake V, Hing CB. Minimally invasive versus conventional exposure for total hip arthroplasty: a systematic review and meta-analysis of clinical and radiological outcomes. Int Orthop 2011;35(2):173–84.

46. Hernandez-Vaquero D, Noriega-Fernandez A, Suarez-Vazquez A. Total knee arthroplasties performed with a mini-incision or a standard incision. Similar results at six months follow-up. BMC Musculoskelet Disord 2010;11:27.

47. Park J-W, Kim Y-H. Simultaneous cemented and cementless total knee replacement in the same patients: a prospective comparison of long-term outcomes using an identical design of NexGen prosthesis. J Bone Joint Surg Br 2011;93(11):1479–86.

48. Harato K, Bourne RB, Victor J, et al. Midterm comparison of posterior cruciate-retaining versus -substituting total knee arthroplasty using the Genesis II prosthesis. A multicenter prospective randomized clinical trial. The Knee 2008;15(3):217–21.

49. Burnett RSJ, Boone JL, Mccarthy KP, et al. A prospective randomized clinical trial of patellar resurfacing and nonresurfacing in bilateral TKA. Clin Orthop Relat Res 2007;PAP:8.

50. Nizard RS, Biau D, Porcher R, et al. A meta-analysis of patellar replacement in total knee arthroplasty. Clin Orthop Relat Res 2005;Mar(432):196–203.

51. Mayman D. Resurfacing versus not resurfacing the patella in total knee arthroplasty 8- to 10-year results. J Arthroplasty 2003;18(5):541–5.

52. Burnett RS, Haydon CM, Rorabeck CH, et al. The John Insall Award: patella resurfacing versus nonresurfacing in total knee arthroplasty. Clin Orthop Relat Res 2004;428:12–25.

53. Gioe TJ, Bowman KR. A randomized comparison of all-polyethylene and metal-backed tibial components. Clin Orthop Relat Res 2000;(380):108–15.

54. Hui C, Salmon L, Maeno S, et al. Five-year comparison of oxidized zirconium and cobalt-chromium femoral components in total knee arthroplasty: a randomized controlled trial. J Bone Joint Surg 2011;93(7):624–30.

55. Spencer JM, Chauhan SK, Sloan K, et al. Computer navigation versus conventional total knee replacement: no difference in functional results at two years. J Bone Joint Surg Br 2007;89(4):477–80.

56. Harvie P, Sloan K, Beaver RJ. Computer navigation vs conventional total knee arthroplasty five-year functional results of a prospective randomized trial. J Arthroplasty 2012;27(5):667–72.

57. Mahomed NN, Davis AM, Hawker G, et al. Inpatient compared with home-based rehabilitation following primary unilateral total hip or knee replacement: a randomized controlled trial. J Bone Joint Surg 2008;90(8):1673–80.

58. Russell TG, Buttrum P, Wootton R, et al. Rehabilitation after total knee replacement via low-bandwidth telemedicine: the patient and therapist experience. J Telemed Telecare 2004;10(Suppl 1):85–7.

59. Rolfson O, Kärrholm J, Dahlberg LE, et al. Patient-reported outcomes in the Swedish Hip Arthroplasty Register: results of a nationwide prospective observational study. J Bone Joint Surg Br 2011;93(7):867–75.

60. Mancuso CA, Salvati EA, Johanson NA, et al. Patients' expectations and satisfaction with total hip arthroplasty. J Arthroplasty 1997;12(4):387–96.

61. Bourne RB, Chesworth B, Davis A, et al. Comparing patient outcomes after THA and TKA: Is there a difference? Clin Orthop Relat Res 2010;468(2):542–6.

62. Ethgen O, Bruyère O, Richy F, et al. Health-related quality of life in total hip and total knee arthroplasty. A qualitative and systematic review of the literature. J Bone Joint Surg Am 2004;86-A(5):963–74.

63. Clement ND, MacDonald D, Howie CR, et al. The outcome of primary total hip and knee arthroplasty in patients aged 80 years or more. J Bone Joint Surg Br 2011;93(9): 1265–70.
64. Arden NK, Kiran A, Judge A, et al. What is a good patient reported outcome after total hip replacement? Osteoarthr Cartil 2011;19(2):155–62.
65. Rolfson O, Dahlberg LE, Nilsson J-A, et al. Variables determining outcome in total hip replacement surgery. J Bone Joint Surg Br 2009;91(2):157–61.
66. Hossain M, Parfitt DJ, Beard DJ, et al. Does pre-operative psychological distress affect patient satisfaction after primary total hip arthroplasty? BMC Musculoskelet Disord 2011;12:122.
67. Mariconda M, Galasso O, Costa GG, et al. Quality of life and functionality after total hip arthroplasty: a long-term follow-up study. BMC Musculoskelet Disord 2011;12(1): 222.
68. Mauermann WJ, Shilling AM, Zuo Z. A comparison of neuraxial block versus general anesthesia for elective total hip replacement: a meta-analysis. Anesth Analg 2006; 103(4):1018–25.
69. Busch CA, Whitehouse MR, Shore BJ, et al. The efficacy of periarticular multimodal drug infiltration in total hip arthroplasty. Clin Orthop Relat Res 2010;468(8):2152–9.
70. Gurlit S, Reinhardt S, Möllmann M. Continuous spinal analgesia or opioid-added continuous epidural analgesia for postoperative pain control after hip replacement. Eur J Anaesthesiol 2004;21(9):708–14.
71. Howell JR, Garbuz DS, Duncan CP. Minimally invasive hip replacement: rationale, applied anatomy, and instrumentation. Orthop Clin North Am 2004;35(2):107–18.
72. Orozco FR, Ong A, Rothman RH. The role of minimally invasive hip surgery in reducing pain. Instructional course lectures 2007;56:121–4.
73. Mahmood A, Zafar MS, Majid I, et al. Minimally invasive hip arthroplasty: a quantitative review of the literature. Br Med Bull 2007;84:37–48.
74. Vresilovic EJ, Hozack WJ, Rothman RH. Incidence of thigh pain after uncemented total hip arthroplasty as a function of femoral stem size. J Arthroplasty 1996;11(3): 304–11.
75. Pour AE, Parvizi J, Sharkey PF, et al. Minimally invasive hip arthroplasty: what role does patient preconditioning play? J Bone Joint Surg Am 2007;89(9):1920–7.
76. McGregor AH, Rylands H, Owen A, et al. Does preoperative hip rehabilitation advice improve recovery and patient satisfaction? J Arthroplasty 2004;19(4):464–8.
77. Iversen MD, Chudasama N, Losina E, et al. Influence of self-reported limb length discrepancy on function and satisfaction 6 years after total hip replacement. J Geriatr Phys Ther 2011;34(3):148–52.
78. Mancuso CA, Graziano S, Briskie LM, et al. Randomized trials to modify patients' preoperative expectations of hip and knee arthroplasties. Clin Orthop Relat Res 2008;466(2):424–31.

Patient-Reported Outcomes for Total Hip and Knee Arthroplasty
Commonly Used Instruments and Attributes of a "Good" Measure

Natalie J. Collins, PhD, PT[a], Ewa M. Roos, PhD, PT[b],*

KEYWORDS

- Total hip arthroplasty • Total knee arthroplasty • Patient-reported outcomes
- Pain • Physical function

KEY POINTS

- Total hip arthroplasty (THA) and total knee arthroplasty (TKA) are well recognized as effective surgical interventions for relieving pain and improving physical function in patients with end-stage degenerative joint disease. Optimization of surgical outcomes requires selection of suitable patients, as well as regular postoperative evaluation utilizing appropriate patient-reported outcome measures.
- Clinicians should consider a number of factors when selecting an appropriate patient-reported instrument for use in THA and TKA patients. These include the specific dimensions measured; administrative burden; accessibility to clinicians and patients; and the psychometric properties of the instrument, such as reliability, validity, and responsiveness to change.
- Based on data acquired in THA and TKA patients for the instruments reviewed, it appears that osteoarthritis-specific and arthroplasty-specific measures for which patients have been involved in the developmental process (HOOS, KOOS, WOMAC, Oxford Hip and Knee Scores) can more consistently be considered "good" patient-reported outcomes for THA and TKA.

THE IMPORTANCE OF APPROPRIATE OUTCOME MEASURES FOR TOTAL JOINT ARTHROPLASTY

Total joint arthroplasty (TJA) is well recognized as an effective surgical intervention for relieving pain and improving physical function associated with end-stage degenerative

Dr. Collins received funding from the National Health and Medical Research Council (Australia) Health Professional Research Training (Post-Doctoral) Fellowship.

Dr. Roos is the developer of the KOOS, HOOS, HAGOS, FAOS, and RAOS. Instruments have been developed in an academic context. Instruments are freely available and no license is required for their use, either academic or commercial. No funding from commercial parties or nonprofit organizations has been received.

[a] Departments of Mechanical Engineering and Physiotherapy, The University of Melbourne, Victoria 3010, Australia; [b] Research Unit for Musculoskeletal Function and Physiotherapy, Institute of Sports Science and Clinical Biomechanics, University of Southern Denmark, Campusvej 55, DK-5230, Odense M, Denmark

* Corresponding author.

E-mail address: eroos@health.sdu.dk

joint disease, such as osteoarthritis (OA). Developed countries commonly report TJA as the most frequent elective surgical procedure. Population-based studies conducted in Scandinavia and Australia reveal a prevalence of total hip arthroplasty (THA) and total knee arthroplasty (TKA) ranging from 61 to 131/100,000,[1] while the lifetime prevalence of THA or TKA in the United Kingdom in 2002 was 6% for females and 5% for males.[2] Importantly, there has been up to a fivefold increase in the rate of THA and TKA over the past two to three decades,[1] with one study projecting a 40-fold increase in THA by 2030.[3] Considering the aging population, growing rates of physical inactivity and obesity, and a subsequent increasing prevalence of symptomatic osteoarthritis,[4] it is not surprising that TJA rates will continue to rise accordingly, resulting in substantial public health expenditure.

To optimize surgical outcomes, it is important that appropriate patients are selected for TJA, and that outcomes are evaluated on an ongoing basis.[5] This is essential given the substantial personal burden, financial costs, and potential surgical and postoperative risks associated with TJA, and that not all patients experience improvements in their condition or are satisfied after surgery.[6] Patient selection for TJA is generally via recommendation by orthopaedic surgeons, primarily on the basis of pain and disability,[7] as well as radiographic progression of joint disease. Indeed, those who have been recommended for THA or TKA by an orthopaedic surgeon tend to report higher levels of preoperative pain and dysfunction.[8] However, in attempting to identify criteria for TJA, there is considerable overlap in levels of pain and dysfunction between those who are and are not recommended for surgery.[8] As such, although pain, disability, and radiographic progression of joint disease are important considerations, there may be other factors that determine patient suitability for TJA, including age, gender, and treatment preferences.[8]

Importantly, appropriate measures that evaluate whether potential gains outweigh costs associated with TJA are vital. Until recently, outcome was commonly defined by rates of surgical complications, morbidity, revision, and mortality,[9] or using surgeon-rated scales that tend to be associated with higher success rates.[6] However, patient-reported outcomes are increasingly used as complements to hard endpoints (such as revision) to evaluate the success of TJA in clinical practice and research. Patient-reported outcomes are measures in which the patient provides an evaluation of his or her health condition or treatment from their perspective.[10] Not only does this minimize observer bias, but it also captures a clearer picture of outcome based on factors that are likely to be important to the patient for whom the surgery was performed.

There are a number of considerations when determining appropriate patient-reported outcomes for use in patients undergoing THA or TKA. Most important is whether the instrument evaluates dimensions that are relevant for such patients, that is, they have high content validity. Evaluation of patients' reasons for undergoing TJA, as well as their postoperative expectations, provides important insight as to dimensions that are important to assess. It appears that the primary reason for TJA is to relieve pain associated with end-stage joint disease, with 98% of those awaiting TKA expecting to experience much less or less pain postoperatively.[11] Other reasons for undergoing TJA are to improve physical function and quality of life (QoL).[11,12] As such, appropriate patient-reported outcomes should capture pain; other symptoms such as stiffness, physical function, and QoL; and perhaps the impact of the patient's condition on mental and emotional well-being. However, many patient-reported outcomes commonly used for TJA fail to address relevant areas, such as activity, participation, and environment,[13] which may limit their use in this cohort.

The second consideration is the measurement, or psychometric, properties of patient-reported outcomes, which may impact results of assessment.[14] Thus, it is important to consider known measurement properties of instruments specific to THA and TKA, such as whether they are repeatable (reliable), whether they measure what they are intended to measure (valid), and whether they are sensitive enough to detect change in a patient's condition postoperatively (responsive). Measures for which little is known regarding their measurement attributes in THA and TKA should be considered with this in mind until such attributes are known. Clinicians also need to be aware of other factors that indicate whether a patient-reported outcome is appropriate for TJA patients. These may include the patient group that it was intended to measure, how easy it is for patients to complete and clinicians to score, and whether the measure is accessible for all patients (eg, language translations) and clinicians (eg, costs associated with utilization).

In considering what constitutes an ideal patient-reported outcome for THA and TKA, the objectives of this review are to:

1. Outline attributes of patient-reported outcomes to consider when selecting measures for THA and TKA patients.
2. Describe patient-reported outcomes that are commonly used to evaluate THA and TKA patients, in terms of their purpose, application, and known measurement properties, in the context of what makes them ideal outcome measures for THA and TKA.

IMPORTANT ATTRIBUTES OF PATIENT-REPORTED OUTCOMES FOR THA AND TKA

As an increasing number of patient-reported outcomes are published and utilized in clinical practice and research, it is vital that decisions regarding which one to use are based on specific attributes. Importantly, given that reported attributes can differ according to the population studied, these should be considered as measured in the intended population. As such, this article focuses on how these attributes apply to patients who have undergone THA and TKA, and where possible draw on data specifically obtained from THA and TKA patients. **Table 1** provides a brief description of attributes that are important to consider when selecting a patient-reported measure for patients undergoing THA and TKA, including definitions of each attribute and appropriate references.

CONSIDERATIONS FOR WHAT CONSTITUTES A "GOOD" PATIENT-REPORTED OUTCOME FOR THA AND TKA

There are a growing number of patient-reported outcomes that can be used to evaluate TJA. A recent systematic review identified 28 instruments that have been used in published studies on rehabilitation after THA and TKA.[15] The current review evaluates 11 of these instruments, which were selected based on the frequency of their use in research[15] and clinical practice, as well as their relevance to THA and TKA patients. This review provides clinicians with a guide as to their suitability for use in TJA patients based on their characteristics (**Table 2**) and psychometric properties (**Table 3** and **Fig. 1**). The included instruments can be classified as (1) disease-specific (or OA-specific) measures (Hip Dysfunction and Osteoarthritis Outcome Score [HOOS], HOOS physical function short form [HOOS-PS], Knee Injury and Osteoarthritis Outcome Score [KOOS], KOOS physical function short form [KOOS-PS], Western Ontario and McMaster Universities Osteoarthritis Index [WOMAC]); (2) intervention-specific (or TJA-specific) measures (Harris Hip Score, Oxford Hip Score, Oxford Knee Score); and (3) generic measures (EQ-5D, Short Form-12 (SF-12), Short

Table 1
Important attributes of patient-reported outcomes for total hip and knee arthroplasty

Attribute	Definition and Rationale for Importance
Intended patient group	The specific patient group for which the instrument was designed. This may be condition specific (eg, OA), intervention specific (eg, THA or TKA), or generic (intended for use in a variety of patients). This will indicate how relevant the instrument is for THA or TKA patients.
Content validity	Whether the instrument contains specific dimensions, subscales (eg, pain, stiffness, function, QoL), items, or questions that are relevant for THA or TKA patients. Defined as present if patients were involved in the development or selection of included items.[18]
Method of administration	Whether the instrument was intended for completion by the patient, or administration by an interviewer or clinician. This also refers to the format in which the measure is delivered (eg, paper-based or online questionnaire; in-person or telephone interview). This has implications for how the measure should be applied to patients, particularly because psychometric properties may have been tested in a particular format.
Respondent burden	Considers the burden on patients completing the measure. Takes into account the number of items patients need to answer and the time taken to complete, as well as how far back patients need to recall to answer particular items.
Administration burden	Considers the burden on clinicians who are administering the measure, such as how long it takes to score, and whether any particular equipment or scoring manuals are required.
Accessibility	How the measure can be obtained for clinical and research use, and whether any fees are applicable. In addition, whether the measure has been translated into languages other than English, and whether any studies have evaluated the validity of cultural adaptations.
Floor and ceiling effects	Floor and ceiling effects refer to whether patients score the lowest and highest possible values, respectively, for a particular measure or subscale. This has implications for being able to show worsening over time if patients have reached the floor of the scale, and improvements over time in those who have reached the ceiling. Floor effects are considered to be acceptable if <15% of patients score the lowest possible score, and ceiling effects acceptable if <15% of patients achieve the highest possible score.[18]
Test-retest reliability	Considers the stability of the instrument, or whether the same result can be obtained on repeated administrations of the measure, when no change in the patient's condition has occurred.[48] Considering the responsiveness (effect size) and within-group variation (standard deviation) commonly seen in TJA, test–retest reliability is considered sufficient if ICC ≥0.75 (for groups of patients) and ≥0.9 (for individual patients).[46,47]
Internal consistency	Assesses how well the items within an instrument or a subscale measure the same characteristic.[48] It is considered adequate if Cronbach's α is ≥0.7.[57]

(continued on next page)

Table 1 (continued)	
Attribute	**Definition and Rationale for Importance**
Construct validity	Refers to the degree to which an instrument measures a particular theoretical construct.[48] It is considered adequate if higher correlations are found with existing measures that assess similar (convergent) constructs (convergent validity), and lower correlations with existing measures that assess dissimilar (divergent) constructs (divergent validity).[18]
Responsiveness	The ability of a measure to detect change in a patient's condition over time.[48] Can be presented as effect size (ES) or standardized response mean (SRM). The SRM takes into account the variability in the change over time, rather than the variability in the baseline measures as per ES. Either can be interpreted as small if <0.5, moderate if 0.5–0.8, and large if >0.8.[58]
Minimal important change (MIC)	The change in score on a patient-reported outcome that represents a meaningful change to the patient in his or her health status.[52,59] This has implications regarding the interpretation of change scores in an instrument; to be confident that a patient has experienced a true improvement in his or her condition, the patient's change score should exceed the MIC. The MIC in turn should exceed the smallest (statistically) detectable difference.
Patient-acceptable symptom state (PASS)	The smallest score beyond which patients would consider themselves to have an acceptable level of symptoms.[60] This is complementary to the MIC, and represents a state of wellness or acceptable baseline level of symptoms, rather than an improvement or change over time. As such, when interpreting effects of an intervention, clinicians must look at the overall improvement or change, but also whether this change brings the patient to an acceptable level (PASS).

Form-36 (SF-36). It should be noted that the disease- and intervention-specific measures have more published data regarding their psychometric properties in TJA, and hence greater weighting is given to discussion of these within relevant sections.

What Patients and Situations was the Instrument Intended for?

Information regarding the intended patient group of an instrument will give clinicians a preliminary indication of its relevance to THA and TKA patients. With respect to the OA-specific instruments, the WOMAC was intended for use in patients with hip or knee OA. The HOOS and KOOS were developed as extensions of the WOMAC to improve content validity for younger or more active patients with posttraumatic OA and preceding injuries of the hip and knee, respectively, and each contain the WOMAC 3.0 items in their entirety. Furthermore, the HOOS-PS and KOOS-PS were derived from HOOS and KOOS subscales of Activities of Daily Living (ADL) and Sport and Recreation Function using item response theory. They were designed as physical function short-form scales, to be used in combination with measures of pain and structural outcomes in patients with hip or knee OA.[16] The intervention-specific instruments were all developed specifically for use in THA patients (Harris Hip Score, Oxford Hip Score) and TKA patients (Oxford Knee Score). In contrast, the generic measures were intended for use across a variety of patient populations. The EQ-5D, which is also frequently used as a utility measure, and the SF-36 were developed

Table 2
Description of commonly used patient-reported outcomes for total hip and knee arthroplasty

Instrument	Content/Dimensions Evaluated; Intended Populations	Method of Administration	Respondent Burden (number of items; recall period; time to complete)	Administration Burden (time to score; equipment required)	Score Interpretation	How to Obtain	Available Language Translations
Disease-specific measures							
HOOS (hip)	Pain, symptoms, ADL, sport/rec, QoL; posttraumatic hip OA and preceding conditions	Patient-completed	40 items; previous week; 10 min	10 min using manual scoring sheet, 2–3 min using scoring spreadsheet (Excel file); both available on website	5 subscales; 0–100 (100 = no problems)	Freely available (www.koos.nu)	Developed in English and Swedish simultaneously; linguistically validated versions (step 1) available in Danish and Lithuanian; clinically validated versions (step 1 and 2) available in Dutch, French, German and Korean
HOOS-PS (hip)	Function (ADL, sport/rec); hip OA	Patient-completed	5 items; previous week; 2 min	<5 min; conversion table[61]	Single score; 0–100 (100 = no difficulty)	Freely available (www.koos.nu)	Available in English and Danish; clinically validated version in French

KOOS (knee)	Pain, symptoms, ADL, sport/rec, QoL; posttraumatic knee OA and preceding conditions	Patient-completed	42 items; previous week; 10 min	10 min using manual scoring sheet, 2–3 min using scoring spreadsheet (Excel file); both available on website	5 subscales; 0–100 (100 = no problems)	Freely available (www.koos.nu)	Original version developed concurrently in English and Swedish; available in 29 languages (www.koos.nu); clinically validated for Swedish, Chinese, Dutch, French, Persian, Portuguese, Russian, Singapore English, Thai and Turkish translations
KOOS-PS (knee)	Function (ADL, sport/rec); knee OA	Patient-completed	7 items; previous week; 2 min	<5 min; conversion table [62]	Single score; 0–100 (100 = no difficulty)	Freely available (www.koos.nu)	Available in English and Swedish; clinically validated versions in French and Portuguese

(continued on next page)

Table 2
(continued)

Instrument	Content/Dimensions Evaluated; Intended Populations	Method of Administration	Respondent Burden (number of items; recall period; time to complete)	Administration Burden (time to score; equipment required)	Score Interpretation	How to Obtain	Available Language Translations
WOMAC (hip, knee)	Pain, stiffness, physical function (ADL); knee and hip OA	Patient-completed or interviewer-administered	24 items; previous 48 hours; 5–10 min	5 min; manual or computer calculation	3 subscales; Likert version: pain (0–20), stiffness (0–8), function (0–68); higher scores indicate worse pain, stiffness or function.	http://www.womac.org (licensing and fee information, permission to use)	Available in >80 languages; validated translations for Arabic, Chinese, Dutch, Finnish, German, Hebrew, Italian, Japanese, Korean, Moroccan, Singapore, Spanish, Swedish, Thai and Turkish
Intervention-specific measures (TJA)							
Harris Hip Score	Pain, function (ADL), absence of deformity, range of motion; total hip replacement	Clinician-administered	10 items; not defined; 5 min	Manual calculation[19]	Single score; 0–100 (90–100 = excellent; 80–90 = good; 70–79 = fair; <70 = poor; categories are an arbitrary classification, not validated.	Available in original publication[19]	No validated translations

Oxford Hip Score	Pain, physical function (ADL); total hip replacement	Patient-completed	12 items; previous 4 weeks; 2–15 min	<5 min; manual calculation	Single score; 0–48 (higher scores = better outcomes)	Freely available (http://phi.uhce.ox.ac.uk/ox_scores.php)	Validated translations in Dutch, Japanese, German and French; widely used in other languages
Oxford Knee Score	Pain, physical function (ADL); total knee replacement	Patient-completed	12 items; previous 4 weeks; 5–10 min	<5 min; manual calculation	Single score; 0–48 (higher scores = better outcomes)	Freely available (http://phi.uhce.ox.ac.uk/ox_scores.php)	Translated and validated in many languages, including Chinese, German, Japanese, Swedish and Thai
Generic measures						
EQ-5D	Mobility, self-care, usual activity, pain/distress, depression/anxiety; intended for use in multiple populations	Patient-completed	6 items; today; <2 min	5 min for simple scoring, longer for conversion to index values; manual calculation using EQ-5D User Guide (website)	5 numbers representing 5 health states; 1–5 (lower scores = better health states); VAS scored 0–100 (100 = best health imaginable)	Available at: http://www.euroqol.org; submit registration form for use.	102 official self-complete official language versions; 62 awaiting ratification (http://www.euroqol.org/eq-5d/eq-5d-products/eq-5d-3l-translations.html)

(continued on next page)

Table 2
(continued)

Instrument	Content/Dimensions Evaluated; Intended Populations	Method of Administration	Respondent Burden (number of items; recall period; time to complete)	Administration Burden (time to score; equipment required)	Score Interpretation	How to Obtain	Available Language Translations
SF-12	Physical functioning, physical role, bodily pain, general health, vitality, social functioning, emotional role, mental health; intended for use in multiple populations	Patient-completed or interviewer-administered	12 items; available in 1-week and 4-week recall versions; 2–3 min	Manual calculation possible, computerized scoring algorithms available (purchase)	8 subscales; 0–100 (higher scores indicate better health)	Available at http://www.qualitymetric.com (annual licensing fee)	Original version in English and Arabic; translation into >50 languages yielded from SF-36 translations (http://www.sf-36.org/tools/sf12.shtml)
SF-36	Physical functioning, physical role, bodily pain, general health, vitality, social functioning, emotional role, mental health; intended for use in multiple populations	Patient-completed or interviewer-administered	36 items; available in 1-week and 4-week recall versions; 7–10 min patient-completed, 16–17 min interviewer-administered	Manual calculation possible, computerised scoring algorithms available (purchase)	8 subscales; 0–100 (higher scores indicate better health)	Original version freely available (http://www.rand.org/health/surveys_tools/mos/mos_core_36item_survey.html); revised version available at: http://www.qualitymetric.com (annual licensing fee)	Original version in English and Arabic; revised version translated into >50 languages (http://www.iqola.org/countries.aspx)

Abbreviation: VAS, visual analogue scale.

Table 3
Psychometric properties of commonly used patient-reported outcomes for total hip and knee arthroplasty, using data from studies in these populations

PRO	Acceptability		Reliability/Repeatability		Validity	
	Floor Effects (>15% have worst possible score)	Ceiling Effects (>15% have best possible score)	Test-Retest (ICC or weighted $\kappa \geq 0.75$ for groups, ≥ 0.9 for individuals)	Internal Consistency (Cronbach's $\alpha \geq 0.7$)	Content Validity (patient involvement during development)	Construct Validity (expected correlations found in comparison with other instruments)
Disease-specific measures						
HOOS: hip[53,63,64]	Pre-op: sport/rec subscale Post-op: no	Pre-op: no 6 months post-op: pain subscale	ADL: groups ✓, individuals ✓ Pain, symptoms, sport/rec, QoL: groups ✓, individuals ✗	✓	✓	✓
HOOS-PS: hip[65,66]	?	?	Groups ✓, individuals ✗	✓	✓	✓
KOOS: knee[25,27,30,67,68]	Pre-op: sport/rec subscale	≤12 months post-op: pain, sport/rec and QoL subscales	Pain, symptoms: groups ✓, individuals ✓ ADL, sport/rec, QoL: groups ✓, individuals ✗	✓	✓	✓
KOOS-PS: knee[62,65,66]	?	?	Groups ✓, individuals ✗	✓	✓	✓

(continued on next page)

Table 3
(continued)

PRO	Acceptability		Reliability/Repeatability		Validity	
	Floor Effects (>15% have worst possible score)	Ceiling Effects (>15% have best possible score)	Test-Retest (ICC or weighted κ ≥0.75 for groups, ≥0.9 for individuals)	Internal Consistency (Cronbach's α ≥0.7)	Content Validity (patient involvement during development)	Construct Validity (expected correlations found in comparison with other instruments)
WOMAC: hip[32,37,39,40,55,69–74]	Pre-op: no Post-op: no	Pre-op: no 1–10 years post-op: pain and stiffness subscales	Patient-completed: Function: groups ✓, individuals ✓ Pain, stiffness: groups ✓, individuals ✗ Interviewer-administered: Pain, function: groups ✓, individuals ✗ Stiffness: groups ✗, individuals ✗	✓	✓	✓
WOMAC: knee[32,35,40,56,73,75–78]	Pre-op: stiffness subscale Post-op: no	Pre-op: stiffness subscale Post-op: pain, stiffness and function subscales	Function: groups ✓, individuals ✓ Pain, stiffness: groups ✓, individuals ✗	✓	✓	✓
Intervention-specific measures						
Harris Hip Score[72,74,79–82]	Pre-op: ? Post-op: no	Pre-op: ? Post-op: yes	Groups ✓, individuals ✗	?	✗	✓

Oxford Hip Score[70,71,83-87]	Pre-op: no Post-op: no	Pre-op: no Post-op: no	Groups ✓, individuals ✓	✓	✓
Oxford Knee Score[77,88-92]	Pre-op: no Post-op: no	Pre-op: no 6 and 12 months post-op: yes	Groups ✓, individuals ✓	✓	✓
Generic measures					
EQ-5D: hip[71]	Pre-op: no Post-op: no	Pre-op: no 1 year post-op: yes (single index)	Groups ?, individuals ?	✗	✓
EQ-5D: knee[76]	Pre-op: no	Pre-op: no	Groups ?, individuals ?	✗	?
SF-12: hip[70,71]	Pre-op: no 1 year post-op: no	Pre-op: no 1 year post-op: no	Physical, mental: groups ?, individuals ?	✗	✓
SF-12: knee[77,93]	Pre-op: no 6 months post-op: no	Pre-op: no 6 months post-op: no	Physical: groups ✓, individuals ✗ Mental: groups ✓, individuals ✓	✗	✓

(continued on next page)

Table 3
(continued)

PRO	Acceptability		Reliability/Repeatability		Validity	
	Floor Effects (>15% have worst possible score)	Ceiling Effects (>15% have best possible score)	Test-Retest (ICC or weighted κ ≥0.75 for groups, ≥0.9 for individuals)	Internal Consistency (Cronbach's α ≥0.7)	Content Validity (patient involvement during development)	Construct Validity (expected correlations found in comparison with other instruments)
SF-36: hip[55,71,74,94,95]	Pre-op: PF, RP, BP, RE 6 months post-op: RP, RE 1 year post-op: RP, RE 2 years post-op: RP 5 years post-op: RP, RE	Pre-op: SF, RE 6 months post-op: RP, BP, SF, RE, MH 1 year post-op: BP, RP, RE, SF 2 years post-op: RP, BP, SF, RE 5 years post-op: RP, BP, SF, RE, MH	Interviewer-administered: PF, BP, MH: groups ✓, individuals ✗ RP, VT, SF, GH, RE: groups ✗, individuals ✗	✓	✗	✓
SF-36: knee[56,75,76,93,94]	Pre-op: PF, RP, RE 6 months post-op: RP, RE 2 years post-op: RP, RE 5 years post-op: RP, RE	Pre-op: RE, SF 6 months post-op: RP, BP, SF, RE, MH 2 years post-op: RP, BP, SF, RE 5 years post-op: RP, BP, SF, RE, MH	PF, BP, GH, SF, MH: groups ✓, individuals ✗ RP, VT, RE: groups ✗, individuals ✗	✓	✗	✓

Abbreviations: BP, bodily pain; GH, general health; MH, mental health; PF, physical functioning; RE, emotional role; RP, physical role; SF, social functioning; VT, vitality.

Tick (✓) indicates adequate measurement properties, cross (✗) indicates unsatisfactory measurement properties, and question mark (?) denotes measurement properties not determined in total hip and knee arthroplasty populations.

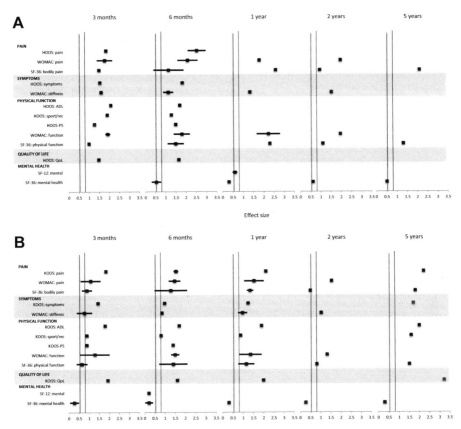

Fig. 1. Five-year responsiveness (effect size, standardized response mean) of commonly used patient-reported outcomes after total hip arthroplasty (A) and total knee arthroplasty (B). (*Data from* Refs.[27,32,35,40,53,55,56,65,66,68,70,71,74,76,83,87,94,96–102])

originally, while the SF-12 was developed as a short-form version of the SF-36. As such, the intervention-specific measures are likely to be most relevant for THA and TKA patients, whereas the disease-specific measures will also be relevant for OA patients of different stages, including those awaiting or undergoing TJA.

What Dimensions Do the Instruments Measure, and are They Relevant to THA and TKA Patients?

Across the OA-specific, TJA-specific, and generic measures, all of the instruments reviewed evaluate physical function with respect to daily activities. In addition, the HOOS, HOOS-PS, KOOS and KOOS-PS also address higher level activity in the form of sport and recreation function. With the exception of the function-specific HOOS-PS and KOOS-PS, the instruments all evaluate pain. The OA-specific measures also evaluate other symptoms such as stiffness (HOOS, KOOS, WOMAC) and swelling, noise, mechanical symptoms, and range of motion (HOOS, KOOS). QoL is most commonly evaluated in the generic measures (EQ-5D, SF-12, SF-36), but has also been incorporated in the OA-specific HOOS and KOOS. Mental and emotional health is evaluated exclusively by the generic instruments. Because the OA- and TJA-specific instruments were designed for individuals with hip/knee OA or those undergoing THA or TKA, their content is likely to reflect dimensions important to those undergoing THA and/or TKA. In comparison, the EQ-5D, SF-12, and SF-36 cover a broader range of items and subscales to reflect their intended use across multiple populations. As such, these generic instruments are less specific for THA and TKA patients when compared to the OA- and TJA-specific instruments. Although this means that they are often less discriminative or responsive when applied to specific patient groups (eg, THA, TKA; **Fig. 1**), they are often well suited to compare populations across conditions, to evaluate aspects of mental and emotional health, and to investigate cost utility of interventions. It has been suggested that a combination of a disease-specific and a generic patient-reported outcome is desirable for a more complete evaluation of OA patients.[17]

For patient-reported outcomes, content validity relates to whether the instrument contains items that are relevant for THA or TKA patients, and is considered present when appropriate patients (ie, hip or knee OA, patients who have undergone THA/TKA) were involved in the development or selection of included items.[18] All of the OA-specific measures are considered to have content validity (**Table 3**). Of the TJA-specific measures, the Oxford Hip and Knee Scores both have content validity, in that patients were involved in item generation and initial testing. In comparison, the Harris Hip Score did not utilize patients in its development and thus content validity cannot be assumed. This is also the case for the three generic instruments, which, by their nature, did not utilize OA or TJA patients specifically in their development. Although they do not assess specific complaints related to hip and knee OA, their items may reflect other aspects such as pain and physical function that are relevant for most adults, including THA or TKA patients.

How was the Instrument Designed to Be Administered?

Eight of the 11 instruments were designed to be completed by the patient, which is an ideal format for a patient-reported outcome. The WOMAC, SF-12, and SF-36 can be patient completed or administered by an interviewer (eg, clinician), which may be useful in situations in which a patient cannot complete the questionnaire him- or herself (eg, visual impairment, other disability). The Harris Hip Score combines patient- and clinician-reported information,[19] which has implications for implementation of the measure, as well as the introduction of observer bias. A modified version of the Harris Hip Score has been developed, which can be administered as a patient-completed tool owing to removal of clinician-reported components of range of motion and deformity.[20] Although this version should be considered where patient completion is desirable, its psychometric properties in TJA are poorly established. As such, and given the greater frequency with which the original Harris Hip Score is used in TJA research and clinical practice, this review focuses on the original version.

How Burdensome is the Instrument for Patients to Complete?

With respect to respondent burden, there are a number of factors to consider. First are the number of items or questions that the instrument contains, the complexity of the items, and the time taken to complete them. Of the instruments reviewed, the number of items varies considerably, from 5 to 42 (**Table 2**). This has implications for the time taken to complete, which may be up to 10 to 15 minutes for instruments that contain more items or ask questions that are more complex in their content or wording. For patients for whom long questionnaires may be onerous, the HOOS-PS and KOOS-PS can be used to substitute the HOOS or KOOS ADL and Sport and Recreation Function subscales, reducing the number of items relating to physical function from 21 to 5 for the hip, and from 22 to 7 for the knee. Furthermore, the instruments vary in the time period that the question refers to (eg, pain over the previous day, week, month). Longer recall periods require patients to remember their conditions over longer periods of time, which may be more difficult for older patients or those with cognitive impairment. However, longer recall may be more desirable for chronic disease such as OA to capture a typical pattern of their condition. A suitable compromise may be an instrument that measures the condition over a week-long period (eg, HOOS, KOOS, acute versions of SF-12 and SF-36). Importantly, the clinician needs to consider the content of the instrument alongside the respondent burden, to ensure that the desired information is obtained without excessively burdening the patient.

How Burdensome is the Instrument for Clinicians to Score?

An important consideration for clinicians selecting a patient-reported outcome is the administration burden, or how easy it is to administer and score. This largely depends on how data are collected, how the instrument is scored, how many items are involved, whether any conversion is required to interpret scores, and whether particular tools are required to derive a score (eg, spreadsheets or formulas). Touch screen scoring reduces administration burden, and when tested yields similar results and psychometric properties to paper-based scoring, suggesting that these administration methods are interchangeable in the clinic.[21,22]

The HOOS and KOOS can be scored manually using instructions provided (10 minutes), or using spread sheets freely available from the website www.koos.nu. These can be used to input and store multiple patient data, and decrease the scoring time to 2 to 3 minutes. Similarly, WOMAC can be scored manually or via a computer spreadsheet obtained from the developers (may involve a fee), but takes approximately 5 minutes as it has fewer items. The HOOS-PS and KOOS-PS can both be scored in less than 5 minutes using supplied conversion tables, while the Oxford Hip and Knee Scores can be calculated as quickly using manual scoring methods. The Harris Hip Score also involves manual calculation, although its inclusion of only 10 items minimizes scoring time. The generic measures involve more in-depth calculations to determine and interpret scores, although scoring algorithms that simplify this process are available from the instrument developers. As such, they may be less desirable for use in a large number of patients or a busy clinical environment.

Is the Instrument Accessible for Clinical Use?

Ideally, an instrument should be easily accessible to clinicians who manage THA and TKA patients. Involvement of financial cost to utilize a given instrument may impact on a clinician's ability to utilize it in his or her practice. The OA- and TJA-specific measures are generally freely available, with the HOOS, HOOS-PS, KOOS, KOOS-PS, Harris Hip Score, and Oxford Hip and Knee Scores obtainable online or in the original publications (see **Table 2** for specific details). However, WOMAC requires users to obtain permission from the developers, and may involve a fee for clinical use. The generic instruments are less accessible, with the EQ-5D requiring registration via the website before use, and the SF-12 and SF-36 involving an annual licensing fee.

Is the Instrument Applicable to Patients from Various Cultural and Language Backgrounds?

A primary consideration regarding accessibility for patients is the languages in which the instrument is available. Language needs will differ for various clinicians depending on their geographic location and their target population. Of the instruments reviewed, all were developed in English (KOOS also developed simultaneously in Swedish). Clinicians working with patients whose first language is not English should first consider those instruments that have linguistically validated and culturally adapted versions available (step 1) that have been subjected to clinical validation to confirm their psychometric properties (step 2).[23] This two-step process takes into account any change in the content of the instrument due to language or cultural differences (eg, use of bath vs shower), and evaluates the psychometric properties of the translated version. Where neither a linguistically or clinically validated translation is available, clinicians should consider that the content and psychometric properties might differ to that of the original instrument. Of the OA- and TJA-specific measures, the KOOS[24–30] and WOMAC[31–44] have undergone the most linguistic and clinical validations. The three generic instruments have also undergone extensive linguistic validation, particularly the EQ-5D,[45] which is not surprising considering their widespread intended use.

Does the Instrument Give the Same Values for the Same Patient on Repeated Administrations?

This refers to the reliability or repeatability of an instrument, and gives an indication of how stable the results are when measuring a patient's unchanged condition on two separate occasions. Clinicians need to consider whether they wish to use the instrument for testing groups of patients (most common) or individual patients. This decision impacts on the acceptable value of reliability that the instrument can demonstrate to be considered sufficiently reliable for the intended purpose (see **Table 1**). On the whole, there has been minimal testing of reliability of the 11 included instruments in THA and TKA cohorts. Instruments with sufficient reliability (intraclass correlation coefficient [ICC] ≥ 0.75[46,47]; **Table 1**) for use in groups of patients undergoing THA are the HOOS (all subscales); HOOS-PS; WOMAC (all subscales); Oxford Hip Score; Harris Hip Score; and SF-36 physical function, bodily pain, and mental health subscales (see **Table 3** for details and references). For groups of patients who have undergone TKA, measures with sufficient reliability are the KOOS (all subscales); KOOS-PS; WOMAC (all subscales); Oxford Knee Score; SF-12 physical and mental subscales; and SF-36 physical function, bodily pain, general health, social function, and mental health subscales (**Table 3**). The reliability of the EQ-5D has not been tested in THA or TKA cohorts. Of the instruments included, only the HOOS ADL subscale, KOOS pain and symptoms subscales, WOMAC function subscale (for THA and TKA patients), Oxford Hip and Knee Scores, and SF-12 mental subscale (for TKA patients) have demonstrated sufficient reliability for use in individual patients (ICC ≥ 0.9[46,47]; **Table 3**). Interestingly, the interviewer-administered version of the WOMAC appears less reliable than the patient-completed version in individuals who have undergone THA (see **Table 3**), which suggests that administrators should utilize the WOMAC in its intended patient-completed format.

Do the Items Within the Instrument Measure Similar Constructs?

The internal consistency of an instrument evaluates how well the items within an instrument or subscale measure the same characteristic[48] (see **Table 1**). This is important to ensure that items proposing to measure the same general construct produce similar scores. The HOOS, HOOS-PS, KOOS, KOOS-PS, WOMAC, Oxford Hip and Knee Scores, and the SF-36 all have adequate internal consistency for use in THA and/or TKA patients (see **Table 3** for details and references). Findings regarding the internal consistency of the Harris Hip Score in THA patients are unclear.

Although the SF-12 has not been evaluated in THA patients, its physical and mental summary components have failed to demonstrate adequate internal consistency in TKA patients. The internal consistency of the EQ-5D has not been evaluated in either THA or TKA patients.

Do the Items Measure What They are Intended to Measure?

Construct validity is a vital psychometric property of any patient-reported outcome, as it represents whether the instrument actually measures what it is intending to measure. As outlined in **Table 1**, this is considered adequate when scores or subscales show higher correlations with existing measures that assess similar constructs, and lower correlations with measures that assess dissimilar constructs.[18] All of the OA- and TJA-specific measures evaluated, as well as the SF-12 and SF-36, have demonstrated expected correlations to other measures when evaluated in THA and/or TKA patients, and are thus considered to have adequate construct validity for use in THA and TKA (see **Table 3** for details and references). Although the EQ-5D appears to measure the expected constructs in THA patients, it is unclear from the published evidence whether this is also the case for TKA patients.

Does the Instrument Have Any Floor or Ceiling Effects?

For clinicians who wish to utilize a patient-reported outcome to evaluate change over time after TJA, any floor or ceiling effects associated with an instrument must be taken into account. Considering the poor status of some patients awaiting TJA, and the generally good postoperative outcomes, preoperative floor effects (patient scoring the worst possible status) and postoperative ceiling effects (patient scoring the best possible status) are more acceptable than vice versa. As such, 15% of patients having the best or worst score is often considered an acceptable cutoff. Instruments or their subscales that have unacceptable floor effects (>15%) may be unable to demonstrate worsening in condition over time, whereas instruments with unacceptable ceiling effects will be unable to show improvement in a patient's condition over time. **Table 3** provides a summary of studies (and references) that have investigated floor and ceiling effects. Of the instruments evaluated, the Oxford Hip Score and SF-12 have shown acceptable floor and ceiling effects before and after THA or TKA (see **Table 3**). On the whole, the OA- and TJA-specific instruments tend to demonstrate acceptable floor effects. The exceptions to these are preoperative scores for the sport and recreation subscale of the HOOS and KOOS, suggesting that this subscale may cover activities that are too high-level for preoperative patients, as well as the stiffness scale of the WOMAC in patients about to undergo TKA. Postoperative ceiling effects, or best possible scores, are more commonly seen (Harris Hip Score, Oxford Knee Score, EQ-5D). This is particularly the case for subscales of pain (HOOS, KOOS, WOMAC), but also for stiffness (WOMAC), function (WOMAC after TKA), and sport and recreation (KOOS) and QoL (KOOS). For TJA patients, the most floor and ceiling effects are seen for the SF-36, which demonstrates similar patterns for THA and TKA patients. Preoperatively, there are unacceptable floor effects largely for the physical subscales (physical function, physical role, bodily pain) as well as for emotional role, whereas preoperative ceiling effects tend to occur for the mental subscales (social functioning, emotional role). Postoperatively, floor effects are consistently seen in the physical role and emotional role subscales, with ceiling effects across a broader spectrum of physical (physical role, bodily pain) and mental (social functioning, emotional role, mental health) subscales. This suggests that some of the subscales included in the SF-36 may be inappropriate or redundant for patients before and after THA or TKA.

Is the Instrument Sensitive Enough to Detect Real Change in a Patient's Condition After TJA?

TJA has a well-established association with improvement in pain and function, particularly in the first 3 to 6 months postoperatively.[6] Reduction in pain typically occurs first, with THA patients reporting pain relief during the first week postoperatively, whereas TKA patients do not report significant pain improvements until up to 6 to 12 weeks after surgery.[49,50] Improvements in physical function tend to occur later, particularly once patients are over the acute postoperative phase.[6,51] As such, patient-reported outcomes need to be sufficiently sensitive to detect improvements in the patient's condition after TJA.

The nature of TJA as an invasive, end-stage intervention that involves a substantial degree of perioperative risk, postoperative morbidity, and financial cost suggests that patient-reported outcomes should be able to detect larger effect sizes (see **Table 1**) to substantiate its use over lower-risk and less expensive interventions such as exercise.[52] Overall, effect size data from published literature reveals that, for both THA and TKA, the OA- and TJA-specific instruments are more responsive at all follow-up times than the generic instruments (see **Fig. 1** for examples and references), which is consistent with previous reports.[6] This suggests that these instruments are more specific for THA and TKA patients, and less influenced by other factors such as comorbidities than the generic instruments, and thus more ideal for use by clinicians to follow up TJA patients.

Figs. 1A (THA) and B (TKA) compare the responsiveness over 5 years of different instruments that evaluate dimensions of pain, symptoms, physical function, QoL, and mental health, and can be used as a quick-reference guide for clinicians wishing to evaluate a particular dimension. To summarize findings for THA on dimensions of pain, symptoms, and physical function, the HOOS, HOOS-PS, and WOMAC tend to be more responsive than the SF-36 at 3 and 6 months. However, there are more inconsistent differences between these measures at longer term follow-ups (1–5 years). It is not possible to compare instruments for QoL, although the HOOS subscale shows large effect sizes at 3 and 6 months after surgery. The two instruments that evaluate mental health, the SF-12 and SF-36, both demonstrate effect sizes that are considered too small after THA (<0.5). As shown in **Fig. 1**B, effect sizes generally tend to be smaller for TKA than THA in the short term. However, data collected 5 years post-TKA show large effect sizes for all dimensions, with the exception of mental health. For pain, the KOOS and WOMAC are consistently more responsive than SF-36 across all follow-up times, whereas for symptoms, the KOOS is more responsive than WOMAC. The KOOS ADL subscale is equivalent to the WOMAC 3.0 function subscale, and these are consequently similarly good in assessing ADL function. The KOOS sport/recreation subscale shows less than adequate effect sizes up until 1 year, with large effect sizes demonstrated at 5 years. As for THA, only the KOOS evaluates QoL, demonstrating consistently large effects, especially 5 years after surgery. Both instruments that evaluate mental health show consistently small or negligible effect sizes.

An important consideration is that the sensitivity of a particular instrument may differ depending on the patient group evaluated. First, some instruments behave differently for THA and TKA patients. This is particularly the case for the WOMAC, which is sensitive to change over 5 years after THA, but has insufficient or questionable sensitivity to change in TKA patients on all subscales at 3 months, and on the stiffness subscale at 1 year after surgery. Similarly, the SF-36 physical subscales are sufficiently sensitive to detect longer-term change after THA, but not

TKA. Second, an instrument's sensitivity may differ according to the age of the patients evaluated. For example, patients aged 66 years or younger show greater responsiveness on all subscales of the HOOS after THA than those aged 67 or older.[53]

What is the Amount of Change That an Instrument Needs to Demonstrate After TJA to Reflect a Meaningful Change to the Patient?

The interpretability of change in patient-reported outcome scores remains difficult. It is not evident that a statistically detectable change is equal to a change considered important to patients. To use patient-reported outcomes as primary outcomes in clinical trials, we need to know the score change that reflects changes in health status that are considered important by patients, and, for the instrument to be useful, this change needs to be greater than the statistically detectable change.[54] The minimal important change (MIC) is the change in score on an instrument that represents a meaningful change to the patient in his or her health status.[52] The recent literature clearly shows that the MIC of an instrument cannot be trusted if determined in one study or by one method only. This is problematic, because in the literature the MIC value of an instrument is often calculated in one (arbitrarily chosen) study and by one method only.[52]

Distribution-based and anchor-based methods can be used to determine the MIC. Most commonly an anchor-based method is applied. Thus the chosen cutoff (a little better, much better, very much better) is of utmost importance. It has been proposed that a higher cutoff should be applied for surgical interventions with a higher risk and cost profile compared to conservative interventions such as exercise; that is, a greater improvement should be required after surgery than after exercise to be considered important to patients. Thus, to be applied in a TJA context, a minimum requirement is that the MIC has been determined in a TJA population.

When five methods were applied to determine the MIC for WOMAC in five populations with OA, large variation was found in MIC values, both across different methods within populations and by the same method across populations.[52] For example, at 6 months after TKA, the two anchor-based methods arrived at MIC values ranging from 13.3 to 42 (scale 0–100), depending on whether the mean change score method or the received operator characteristics method were used, and if absolute or change scores were applied. The corresponding 95% confidence intervals (CIs) were very large, in total ranging from 0.5 to 63. Thus, great caution is needed when interpreting and using published MIC values.[52]

Currently, the MIC has been determined in only a few TJA populations and for only two of the instruments reviewed. The methods used, cutoffs chosen, and time to follow-up may contribute to the variance seen in the few studies performed. With respect to the OA- and TJA-specific measures, the MIC has been determined only for TJA patients for the WOMAC. When calculated in a THA population at 6 and 24 months, the MIC for pain was 29 and 33 on a 0 to 100 scale, respectively; 27 and 33 for function, respectively; and 26 for stiffness at both follow-up times.[55] Slightly lower MIC values have been reported in TKA patients, particularly at 6 months after surgery (pain: 23 at 6 months, 28 at 2 years; stiffness: 15 at 6 months, 21 at 2 years; function: 19 at 6 months, 21 at 2 years).[56] In the study comparing five different methods, the MIC value corresponding to "a little better" for WOMAC at 6 months after TKA was 13.3 (95% CI, 0.5–26.1).[52]

Of the generic instruments, only the SF-36 has MIC values reported after THA and TKA. In patients who are 6 months post-THA, the MIC of the eight SF-36 subscales ranges from 0.4 for general health to 20.4 for physical function (0–100 scale).[55] Similar values have been reported in TKA patients at 6 months (MIC range: 0.9 for general health to 17 for bodily pain).[56] Although these values are compromised by lack of verification from other studies, they do highlight potentially vast differences across the different SF-36 dimensions evaluated. The patient-acceptable symptom state (PASS) has not been evaluated for any of the reviewed instruments in THA and TKA patients.

SUMMARY

Although the effectiveness of THA and TKA as interventions for end-stage degenerative joint disease has been well established, the use of instruments that measure outcome from the patient's perspective are relatively poorly investigated. Considering the increasing prevalence, associated risks, and high personal and financial cost associated with THA and TKA, patient-reported outcomes are required to ensure optimal selection of patients, and that postoperative outcomes outweigh the burden associated with surgical procedures. It is clear from the information presented that clinicians need to consider a number of factors when selecting a "good" patient-reported outcome for use in their TJA patients. Not only does the instrument need to measure dimensions appropriate for THA and TKA patients, but it also needs to have minimal administrative burden, accessibility to a variety of clinicians and patients, reliability, validity, and responsiveness to change. Furthermore, knowledge regarding the minimal score that patients deem to be meaningful is useful in interpreting whether a patient has experienced real improvement in their condition after surgery. It is clear that further studies are required, particularly to fill some of the gaps regarding known psychometric properties of patient-reported outcomes for THA and TKA. Based on data acquired in THA and TKA patients for the instruments reviewed, it appears that OA-specific and TJA-specific measures for which patients have been involved in the developmental process (HOOS, KOOS, WOMAC, Oxford Hip and Knee Scores) can more consistently be considered "good" patient-reported outcomes for THA and TKA. Clinicians wishing to evaluate a broader range of dimensions may choose to complement these with one of the generic measures evaluated, bearing in mind the practical issues and psychometric limitations of these instruments when applied to THA and TKA patients.

REFERENCES

1. Singh JA. Epidemiology of knee and hip arthroplasty: a systematic review. Open Orthop J 2011;5:80–5.
2. Steel N, Melzer D, Gardener E, et al. Need for and receipt of hip and knee replacement—a national population survey. Rheumatology 2006;45:1437–41.
3. Birrell F, Johnell O, Silman A. Projecting the need for hip replacement over the next three decades: influence of changing demography and threshold for surgery. Ann Rheum Dis 1999;58:569–72.
4. Nguyen US, Zhang Y, Zhu Y, et al. Increasing prevalence of knee pain and symptomatic knee osteoarthritis: survey and cohort data. Ann Intern Med 2011; 155:725–32.
5. Wylde V, Blom AW. Assessment of outcomes after hip arthroplasty. Hip Int 2009; 19:1–7.
6. Jones CA, Beaupre LA, Johnston DW, et al. Total joint arthroplasties: current concepts of patient outcomes after surgery. Rheum Dis Clin North Am 2007;33: 71–86.
7. Wright JG, Coyte P, Hawker G, et al. Variation in orthopedic surgeons' perceptions of the indications for and outcomes of knee replacement. CMAJ 1995;152:687–97.

8. Gossec L, Paternotte S, Maillefert JF, et al. The role of pain and functional impairment in the decision to recommend total joint replacement in hip and knee osteoarthritis: an international cross-sectional study of 1909 patients. Report of the OARSI-OMERACT Task Force on total joint replacement. Osteoarthritis Cartilage 2011;19: 147–54.

9. Ahmad MA, Xypnitos FN, Giannoudis PV. Measuring hip outcomes: common scales and checklists. Injury 2011;42:259–64.

10. Patrick DL, Burke LB, Powers JH, et al. Patient-reported outcomes to support medical product labeling claims: FDA perspective. Value Health 2007;10(Suppl 2): S125–37.

11. Nilsdotter AK, Toksvig-Larsen S, Roos EM. Knee arthroplasty: are patients' expectations fulfilled? A prospective study of pain and function in 102 patients with 5-year follow-up. Acta Orthop 2009;80:55–61.

12. Suarez-Almazor ME, Richardson M, Kroll TL, et al. A qualitative analysis of decision-making for total knee replacement in patients with osteoarthritis. J Clin Rheumatol 2010;16:158–63.

13. Alviar MJ, Olver J, Brand C, et al. Do patient-reported outcome measures used in assessing outcomes in rehabilitation after hip and knee arthroplasty capture issues relevant to patients? Results of a systematic review and ICF linking process. J Rehabil Med 2011;43:374–81.

14. Singh JA. Responsiveness differences in outcome instruments after revision hip arthroplasty: what are the implications? BMC Musculoskel Disord 2011;12:107.

15. Alviar MJ, Olver J, Brand C, et al. Do patient-reported outcome measures in hip and knee arthroplasty rehabilitation have robust measurement attributes? A systematic review. J Rehabil Med 2011;43:572–83.

16. Gossec L, Hawker G, Davis AM, et al. OMERACT/OARSI initiative to define states of severity and indication for joint replacement in hip and knee osteoarthritis. J Rheumatol 2007;34:1432–5.

17. Hawker G, Melfi C, Paul J, et al. Comparison of a generic (SF-36) and a disease specific (WOMAC) (Western Ontario and McMaster Universities Osteoarthritis Index) instrument in the measurement of outcomes after knee replacement surgery. J Rheumatol 1995;22:1193–6.

18. Terwee CB, Bot SD, de Boer MR, et al. Quality criteria were proposed for measurement properties of health status questionnaires. J Clin Epidemiol 2007;60:34–42.

19. Harris WH. Traumatic arthritis of the hip after dislocation and acetabular fractures: treatment by mold arthroplasty: An end-result study using a new method of result evaluation. J Bone Joint Surg [Am] 1969;51:737–55.

20. Byrd JW, Jones KS. Prospective analysis of hip arthroscopy with 2-year follow-up. Arthroscopy 2000;16:578–87.

21. Gudbergsen H, Bartels EM, Krusager P, et al. Test-retest of computerized health status questionnaires frequently used in the monitoring of knee osteoarthritis: a randomized crossover trial. BMC Musculoskel Disord 2011;12:190.

22. Theiler R, Spielberger J, Bischoff HA, et al. Clinical evaluation of the WOMAC 3.0 OA Index in numeric rating scale format using a computerized touch screen version. Osteoarthritis Cartilage 2002;10:479–81.

23. Beaton DE, Bombardier C, Guillemin F, et al. Guidelines for the process of cross-cultural adaptation of self-report measures. Spine 2000;25:3186–91.

24. Chaipinyo K. Test-retest reliability and construct validity of Thai version of Knee Osteoarthritis Outcome Score (KOOS). Thai J Phys Ther 2009;31:67–76.

25. de Groot IB, Favejee MM, Reijman M, et al. The Dutch version of the Knee Injury and Osteoarthritis Outcome Score: a validation study. Health Qual Life Outcomes 2008; 6:16.

26. Goncalves RS, Cabri J, Pinheiro JP, et al. Cross-cultural adaptation and validation of the Portuguese version of the Knee Injury and Osteoarthritis Outcome Score (KOOS). Osteoarthritis Cartilage 2009;17:1156–62.

27. Ornetti P, Parratte S, Gossec L, et al. Cross-cultural adaptation and validation of the French version of the Knee Injury and Osteoarthritis Outcome Score (KOOS) in knee osteoarthritis patients. Osteoarthritis Cartilage 2008;16:423–8.

28. Paker N, Bugdayci D, Sabirli F, et al. Knee Injury and Osteoarthritis Outcome Score: reliability and validation of the Turkish version. Turkiye Klinikleri J Med Sci 2007;27: 350–6.

29. Salavati M, Mazaheri M, Negahban H, et al. Validation of a Persian-version of Knee Injury and Osteoarthritis Outcome Score (KOOS) in Iranians with knee injuries. Osteoarthritis Cartilage 2008;16:1178–82.

30. Xie F, Li SC, Roos EM, et al. Cross-cultural adaptation and validation of Singapore English and Chinese versions of the Knee Injury and Osteoarthritis Outcome Score (KOOS) in Asians with knee osteoarthritis in Singapore. Osteoarthritis Cartilage 2006;14:1098–103.

31. Bae SC, Lee HS, Yun HR, et al. Cross-cultural adaptation and validation of Korean Western Ontario and McMaster Universities (WOMAC) and Lequesne osteoarthritis indices for clinical research. Osteoarthritis Cartilage 2001;9:746–50.

32. Escobar A, Quintana JM, Bilbao A, et al. Validation of the Spanish version of the WOMAC questionnaire for patients with hip or knee osteoarthritis. Western Ontario and McMaster Universities Osteoarthritis Index. Clin Rheumatol 2002;21:466–71.

33. Faik A, Benbouazza K, Amine B, et al. Translation and validation of Moroccan Western Ontario and McMaster Universities (WOMAC) osteoarthritis index in knee osteoarthritis. Rheumatol Int 2008;28:677–83.

34. Guermazi M, Poiraudeau S, Yahia M, et al. Translation, adaptation and validation of the Western Ontario and McMaster Universities osteoarthritis index (WOMAC) for an Arab population: the Sfax modified WOMAC. Osteoarthritis Cartilage 2004;12:459–68.

35. Hashimoto H, Hanyu T, Sledge CB, et al. Validation of a Japanese patient-derived outcome scale for assessing total knee arthroplasty: comparison with Western Ontario and McMaster Universities osteoarthritis index (WOMAC). J Orthop Sci 2003;8:288–93.

36. Kuptniratsaikul V, Rattanachaiyanont M. Validation of a modified Thai version of the Western Ontario and McMaster (WOMAC) osteoarthritis index for knee osteoarthri- tis. Clin Rheumatol 2007;26:1641–5.

37. Roorda LD, Jones CA, Waltz M, et al. Satisfactory cross cultural equivalence of the Dutch WOMAC in patients with hip osteoarthritis waiting for arthroplasty. Ann Rheum Dis 2004;63:36–42.

38. Salaffi F, Leardini G, Canesi B, et al. Reliability and validity of the Western Ontario and McMaster Universities (WOMAC) Osteoarthritis Index in Italian patients with osteo- arthritis of the knee. Osteoarthritis Cartilage 2003;11:551–60.

39. Soderman P, Malchau H. Validity and reliability of Swedish WOMAC osteoarthritis index: a self-administered disease-specific questionnaire (WOMAC) versus generic instruments (SF-36 and NHP). Acta Orthop Scand 2000;71:39–46.

40. Soininen JV, Paavolainen PO, Gronblad MA, et al. Validation study of a Finnish version of the Western Ontario and McMasters University osteoarthritis index. Hip Int 2008;18:108–11.

41. Stucki G, Meier D, Stucki S, et al. [Evaluation of a German version of WOMAC (Western Ontario and McMaster Universities) Arthrosis Index]. Z Rheumatol 1996; 55:40–9.
42. Thumboo J, Chew LH, Soh CH. Validation of the Western Ontario and McMaster University osteoarthritis index in Asians with osteoarthritis in Singapore. Osteoarthritis Cartilage 2001;9:440–6.
43. Tuzun EH, Eker L, Aytar A, et al. Acceptability, reliability, validity and responsiveness of the Turkish version of WOMAC osteoarthritis index. Osteoarthritis Cartilage 2005;13:28–33.
44. Wigler I, Neumann L, Yaron M. Validation study of a Hebrew version of WOMAC in patients with osteoarthritis of the knee. Clin Rheumatol 1999;18:402–5.
45. EuroQol Group. Available at: http://www.euroqol.org/eq-5d/eq-5d-products/eq-5d-3l-translations.html. Accessed May 4, 2012.
46. Nunnally JC. Psychometric theory. 2nd edition. New York: McGraw-Hill; 1978.
47. Rosner B. Fundamentals of biostatistics. Belmont, CA: Duxbury Press; 2005.
48. Portney LG, Watkins MP. Foundations of clinical research: applications to practice. 3rd edition. Upper Saddle River, NJ: Prentice Hall; 2009.
49. Aarons H, Hall G, Hughes S, et al. Short-term recovery from hip and knee arthroplasty. J Bone Joint Surg [Br] 1996;78:555–8.
50. Brander VA, Stulberg SD, Adams AD, et al. Predicting total knee replacement pain: a prospective, observational study. Clin Orthop Relat Res 2003:27–36.
51. Fitzgerald JD, Orav EJ, Lee TH, et al. Patient quality of life during the 12 months following joint replacement surgery. Arthritis Rheum 2004;51:100–9.
52. Terwee CB, Roorda LD, Dekker J, et al. Mind the MIC: large variation among populations and methods. J Clin Epidemiol 2010;63:524–34.
53. Nilsdotter AK, Lohmander LS, Klassbo M, et al. Hip disability and osteoarthritis outcome score (HOOS)—validity and responsiveness in total hip replacement. BMC Musculoskel Disord 2003;4:10.
54. Terwee CB, Roorda LD, Knol DL, et al. Linking measurement error to minimal important change of patient-reported outcomes. J Clin Epidemiol 2009;62:1062–7.
55. Quintana JM, Escobar A, Bilbao A, et al. Responsiveness and clinically important differences for the WOMAC and SF-36 after hip joint replacement. Osteoarthritis Cartilage 2005;13:1076–83.
56. Escobar A, Quintana JM, Bilbao A, et al. Responsiveness and clinically important differences for the WOMAC and SF-36 after total knee replacement. Osteoarthritis Cartilage 2007;15:273–80.
57. Streiner DL, Norman GR. Health measurement scales: a practical guide to their development and use. 4th edition. Oxford: Oxford University Press; 2008.
58. Cohen J. Statistical power analysis for the behavioral sciences. 2nd edition. Hillsdale, NJ: Lawrence Erlbaum Associates; 1988.
59. Tubach F, Ravaud P, Baron G, et al. Evaluation of clinically relevant changes in patient reported outcomes in knee and hip osteoarthritis: the minimal clinically important improvement. Ann Rheum Dis 2005;64:29–33.
60. Tubach F, Ravaud P, Baron G, et al. Evaluation of clinically relevant states in patient reported outcomes in knee and hip osteoarthritis: the patient acceptable symptom state. Ann Rheum Dis 2005;64:34–7.
61. Davis AM, Perruccio AV, Canizares M, et al. The development of a short measure of physical function for hip OA HOOS-Physical Function Shortform (HOOS-PS): an OARSI/OMERACT initiative. Osteoarthritis Cartilage 2008;16:551–9.

62. Perruccio AV, Stefan Lohmander L, Canizares M, et al. The development of a short measure of physical function for knee OA KOOS-Physical Function Shortform (KOOS-PS)—an OARSI/OMERACT initiative. Osteoarthritis Cartilage 2008;16:542–50.

63. de Groot IB, Reijman M, Terwee CB, et al. Validation of the Dutch version of the Hip Disability and Osteoarthritis Outcome Score. Osteoarthritis Cartilage 2007;15: 104–9.

64. Ornetti P, Parratte S, Gossec L, et al. Cross-cultural adaptation and validation of the French version of the Hip Disability and Osteoarthritis Outcome Score (HOOS) in hip osteoarthritis patients. Osteoarthritis Cartilage 2010;18:522–9.

65. Davis AM, Perruccio AV, Canizares M, et al. Comparative, validity and responsiveness of the HOOS-PS and KOOS-PS to the WOMAC physical function subscale in total joint replacement for osteoarthritis. Osteoarthritis Cartilage 2009;17:843–7.

66. Ruyssen-Witrand A, Fernandez-Lopez CJ, Gossec L, et al. Psychometric properties of the OARSI/OMERACT osteoarthritis pain and functional impairment scales: ICOAP, KOOS-PS and HOOS-PS. Clin Exp Rheumatol 2011;29:231–7.

67. Roos EM, Roos HP, Lohmander LS, et al. Knee Injury and Osteoarthritis Outcome Score (KOOS)—development of a self-administered outcome measure. J Orthop Sports Phys Ther 1998;28:88–96.

68. Roos EM, Toksvig-Larsen S. Knee injury and Osteoarthritis Outcome Score (KOOS)—validation and comparison to the WOMAC in total knee replacement. Health Qual Life Outcomes 2003;1:17.

69. Bellamy N. WOMAC Osteoarthritis Index User Guide. London, Ontario: Canada. 1995.

70. Garbuz DS, Xu M, Sayre EC. Patients' outcome after total hip arthroplasty: a comparison between the Western Ontario and McMaster Universities index and the Oxford 12-item Hip Score. J Arthroplasty 2006;21:998–1004.

71. Ostendorf M, van Stel HF, Buskens E, et al. Patient-reported outcome in total hip replacement: a comparison of five instruments of health status. J Bone Joint Surg [Br] 2004;86:801–8.

72. Soderman P, Malchau H, Herberts P. Outcome of total hip replacement: a comparison of different measurement methods. Clin Orthop Relat Res 2001:163–72.

73. Stucki G, Sangha O, Stucki S, et al. Comparison of the WOMAC (Western Ontario and McMaster Universities) osteoarthritis index and a self-report format of the self-administered Lequesne-Algofunctional index in patients with knee and hip osteoarthritis. Osteoarthritis Cartilage 1998;6:79–86.

74. Wright JG, Young NL. A comparison of different indices of responsiveness. J Clin Epidemiol 1997;50:239–46.

75. Bombardier C, Melfi C, Paul J, et al. Comparison of a generic and a disease-specific measure of pain and physical function after knee replacement surgery. Med Care 1995;33:AS131–AS144.

76. Brazier J, Harper R, Munro J, et al. Generic and condition-specific outcome measures for people with osteoarthritis of the knee. Rheumatology (Oxford) 1999;38: 870–7.

77. Impellizzeri F, Mannion A, Leunig M, et al. Comparison of the Reliability, Responsiveness, and Construct Validity of 4 Different Questionnaires for Evaluating Outcomes after Total Knee Arthroplasty. J Arthroplasty; 2011;26(6):861–9.

78. Xie F, Li SC, Goeree R, et al. Validation of Chinese Western Ontario and McMaster Universities Osteoarthritis Index (WOMAC) in patients scheduled for total knee replacement. Qual Life Res 2008;17:595–601.

79. Garellick G, Malchau H, Herberts P. Specific or general health outcome measures in the evaluation of total hip replacement: a comparison between the Harris Hip Score and the Nottingham Health Profile. J Bone Joint Surg [Br] 1998;80:600–6.

80. Lieberman JR, Dorey F, Shekelle P, et al. Outcome after total hip arthroplasty. Comparison of a traditional disease-specific and a quality-of-life measurement of outcome. J Arthroplasty 1997;12:639–45.

81. Soderman P, Malchau H. Is the Harris Hip Score system useful to study the outcome of total hip replacement? Clin Orthop Relat Res 2001:189–97.

82. Wamper KE, Sierevelt IN, Poolman RW, et al. The Harris Hip Score: do ceiling effects limit its usefulness in orthopedics? Acta Orthop 2010;81:703–7.

83. Dawson J, Fitzpatrick R, Carr A, et al. Questionnaire on the perceptions of patients about total hip replacement. J Bone Joint Surg [Br] 1996;78:185–90.

84. Fitzpatrick R, Morris R, Hajat S, et al. The value of short and simple measures to assess outcomes for patients of total hip replacement surgery. Qual Health Care 2000;9:146–50.

85. Gosens T, Hoefnagels NH, de Vet RC, et al. The "Oxford Heup Score": the translation and validation of a questionnaire into Dutch to evaluate the results of total hip arthroplasty. Acta Orthop 2005;76:204–11.

86. Naal FD, Sieverding M, Impellizzeri FM, et al. Reliability and validity of the cross-culturally adapted German Oxford Hip Score. Clin Orthop Relat Res 2009;467: 952–7.

87. Uesugi Y, Makimoto K, Fujita K, et al. Validity and responsiveness of the Oxford Hip Score in a prospective study with Japanese total hip arthroplasty patients. J Orthop Sci 2009;14:35–9.

88. Dawson J, Fitzpatrick R, Murray D, et al. Questionnaire on the perceptions of patients about total knee replacement. J Bone Joint Surg [Br] 1998;80:63–9.

89. Haverkamp D, Breugem SJ, Sierevelt IN, et al. Translation and validation of the Dutch version of the Oxford 12-item knee questionnaire for knee arthroplasty. Acta Orthop 2005;76:347–52.

90. Naal F, Impellizzeri F, Sieverding M, et al. The 12-item Oxford Knee Score: cross-cultural adaptation into German and assessment of its psychometric properties in patients with osteoarthritis of the knee. Osteoarthritis Cartilage 2009;17:49–52.

91. Padua R, Zanoli G, Ceccarelli E, et al. The Italian version of the Oxford 12-item Knee Questionnaire—cross-cultural adaptation and validation. Int Orthop 2003;27: 214–6.

92. Xie F, Li S, Lo N, et al. Cross-cultural adaptation and validation of Singapore English and Chinese Versions of the Oxford Knee Score (OKS) in knee osteoarthritis patients undergoing total knee replacement. Osteoarthritis Cartilage 2007;15:1019–24.

93. Dunbar MJ, Robertsson O, Ryd L, et al. Appropriate questionnaires for knee arthroplasty: results of a survey of 3600 patients from The Swedish Knee Arthroplasty Registry. J Bone Joint Surg [Br] 2001;83:339–44.

94. Busija L, Osborne RH, Nilsdotter A, et al. Magnitude and meaningfulness of change in SF-36 scores in four types of orthopedic surgery. Health Qual Life Outcomes 2008;6:55.

95. Mangione CM, Goldman L, Orav EJ, et al. Health-related quality of life after elective surgery: measurement of longitudinal changes. J Gen Intern Med 1997;12:686–97.

96. Davis AM, Lohmander LS, Wong R, et al. Evaluating the responsiveness of the ICOAP following hip or knee replacement. Osteoarthritis Cartilage 2010;18:1043–5.

97. Blanchard C, Feeny D, Mahon JL, et al. Is the Health Utilities Index responsive in total hip arthroplasty patients? J Clin Epidemiol 2003;56:1046–54.

98. Nilsdotter AK, Roos EM, Westerlund JP, et al. Comparative responsiveness of measures of pain and function after total hip replacement. Arthritis Rheum 2001;45: 258–62.

99. Shi HY, Mau LW, Chang JK, et al. Responsiveness of the Harris Hip Score and the SF-36: five years after total hip arthroplasty. Qual Life Res 2009;18:1053–60.

100. Shi HY, Chang JK, Wong CY, et al. Responsiveness and minimal important differences after revision total hip arthroplasty. BMC Musculoskel Disord 2010;11:261.

101. Kirschner S, Walther M, Bohm D, et al. German short musculoskeletal function assessment questionnaire (SMFA-D): comparison with the SF-36 and WOMAC in a prospective evaluation in patients with primary osteoarthritis undergoing total knee arthroplasty. Rheumatol Int 2003;23:15–20.

102. Nilsdotter AK, Toksvig-Larsen S, Roos EM. A 5 year prospective study of patient-relevant outcomes after total knee replacement. Osteoarthritis Cartilage 2009;17: 601–6.

Health-Related Quality of Life After Total Joint Arthroplasty
A Scoping Review

C. Allyson Jones, PT, PhD[a],*, Sheri Pohar, BScPharm, PhD[b]

KEYWORDS

- Joint arthroplasty • Knee arthroplasty • Health status • Recovery

KEY POINTS

- This review examines recovery after total hip and knee arthroplasty. The specific aims are to (1) provide an overview of the different types of disease-specific, generic, and utility outcome measures used to assess recovery after total hip arthroplasty and total knee arthroplasty and (2) summarize the reported changes in health-related quality of life after total joint arthroplasty.
- Of the 1171 citations, 33 articles were included. Disease-specific measures reported large and important changes (assessed both with minimally clinically important differences and effect size criteria), primarily for pain and function over short-term and long-term recovery. Smaller but important changes were reported with generic and utility measures. Changes were largest in the pain and physical function domains.

INTRODUCTION

A primary goal of health care for any chronic disease, including arthritis, is to maintain or improve health-related quality of life (HRQL).[1] A recent shift in the conceptual model of disease has moved from viewing the "consequences of disease" or the impact of health to components of health. Impairment caused by arthritis is reflected by pain and functional limitations and are independent factors that predict the recommendation of total joint arthroplasty.[2]

Although clinical measures have traditionally been the standard to assess outcomes for total joint arthroplasty, there is a consensus that HRQL outcome measures

DISCLOSURE: Dr Sheri Pohar contributed to this work while on leave from Canadian Agency for Drugs and Technologies in Health (CADTH). As such, the views presented in this article do not necessarily represent the views of CADTH. Dr Allyson Jones received salary support from the Alberta Heritage Foundation for Medical Research and the Canadian Institutes of Health Research.

a Department of Physical Therapy, University of Alberta, Rm 2-50, Corbett Hall, Edmonton, AB, Canada T6G 2G4; b Canadian Agency for Drugs and Technologies in Health (CADTH), Suite 1331, 10235 101 Street, Edmonton, AB, Canada T5J 3G1
* Corresponding author.
E-mail address: cajones@ualberta.ca

should be used in the research and clinical settings.[3] HRQL outcomes are validated patient- or proxy-reported outcome measures. Available evidence supports the reliability and validity of HRQL measures in clinical practice; however, uncertainly about clinical usefulness hinders their full adoption into clinical practice.[4]

HRQL is a complex and multidimensional concept that is only one component of overall quality of life. The focus of HRQL measures is on the quality of life attributes that are affected by health. It represents domains that are directly related to the health of a person, including symptoms, mental health, physical functioning, role function- ing, and overall perception of health.[5] The concept of HRQL embodies not only physical components but also psychological and social factors that are viewed as integral components of health.

The evaluation of HRQL in chronic diseases and related interventions requires measures that reflect a broad array of dimensions. In turn, the measurement of HRQL provides clinically valuable information on how arthritis impacts health. HRQL information can be used to assist in the management of patients, for clinical policy, research, health policy, and decision making.

Although the use of HRQL outcomes for total joint arthroplasties in research and clinical settings has increased considerably, to our knowledge the recovery reported with pain and function after total joint arthroplasty has not been systematically summarized in the context of a scoping review. A challenge in summarizing change with HRQL measures used in total joint arthroplasty is the differing psychometric properties of the various measures used.[6] The primary aims of this scoping review were to (1) provide an overview of the different types of disease-specific, generic, and utility measures used to assess recovery after total hip arthroplasty (THA) and total knee arthroplasty (TKA) and (2) summarize the reported change after total joint arthroplasty.

METHODS
Study Design

A scoping review of the literature was conducted using formal methods of review.[7] A scoping review differs from other types of reviews in that it undertakes broader topics, includes different study designs, and does not necessarily assess the quality of the studies. Within this review the results of the included studies were not combined but rather reported individually.

Study inclusion criteria were the following: (1) The study population must have had an elective primary THA or TKA; (2) the study designs must be prospective follow-up or before–after study design with a baseline/preoperative measure and a postoper- ative follow-up; and (3) the study used validated HRQL measures. Studies of patients with unicompartmental, hemiarthroplasties, and hip fractures were excluded. Cohort, case control, and randomized controlled trials published in full were eligible for inclusion. Abstracts, letters, and review articles were excluded.

Search Strategies

Electronic searches of MEDLINE, EMBASE, CINAHL, SPORTDiscus, and EBM Reviews were conducted by a medical librarian using the search terms "total hip replacement," "total knee replacement," "arthroplasty," and "quality of life." The terms were searched as MeSH terms and subject headings and also as "free text" keywords. Retrieval was limited to English publications from January 2001 to November 2011. All duplicate citations were identified and removed. For duplicate studies, only the largest trial was included.

Study Selection

Abstracts were initially screened for relevance by one of three reviewers. The full-text publications of potentially relevant articles were obtained. Second-level screening of full-text studies was performed by two of three reviewers using prespecified inclusion and exclusion criteria. The full-text article was independently reviewed by both reviewers. Disagreement between reviewers about the final inclusion of studies into the scoping review was resolved through consensus. Full-text papers were included only if consensus was achieved by reviewers.

Data Extraction

Study description, patient characteristics, and HRQL outcomes were extracted from the reports by a single reviewer using a standardized data extraction form. A second reviewer independently checked for discrepancies.

Analysis

When the change in HRQL over time was not reported, changes from baseline were calculated for each time point using baseline and postoperative scores. The clinical importance of the observed changes in HRQL before and after total joint arthroplasty was interpreted in comparison to literature based minimally clinically important differences (MCIDs) in orthopaedic surgery where available. The MCID is the smallest difference in the score of a measure in which patients regard as a change.[8] This change in score is clinically important. For measures for which MCIDs specific to total joint arthroplasty were not reported in the literature, population-based thresholds or those specific to another condition were used for comparison purposes.

To standardize mean differences between baseline and postoperative scores and allow comparison among studies, effect sizes were calculated. The effect size quantified the effect of total joint arthroplasty in terms of standard deviation units and estimated the magnitude of change over time. The magnitude of the effect sizes were compared to Cohen's classification (effect sizes of 0.2, 0.5, and 0.8 are considered as small, moderate, and large, respectively).[9] For those studies that did not report the effect sizes but included the mean and standard deviation of the measures for at least two time points, the effect size was calculated as the change from baseline divided by the standard deviation of the baseline scores. Effect sizes could not be calculated for studies that did not report the standard deviation of the baseline scores or reported only median scores.

RESULTS

Of the 1171 citations that were identified, 69 (5.9%) studies were obtained for full-text screening, 33 of which were included in our review (**Fig. 1**). The most frequently reported measures were the Western Ontario and McMaster Universities (WOMAC) Osteoarthritis Index and the SF-36 Health Survey; however, other disease-specific and generic measures were used to evaluate change over the continuum of care for total joint arthroplasty. Most studies in this review were prospective observational studies (n = 29).

Disease-Specific Measures

Because HRQL is a subjective concept, its measurement can be challenging. A taxonomy for health measures identify disease-specific or joint-specific measures for total joint arthroplasty. Disease-specific measures focus on patients with the same

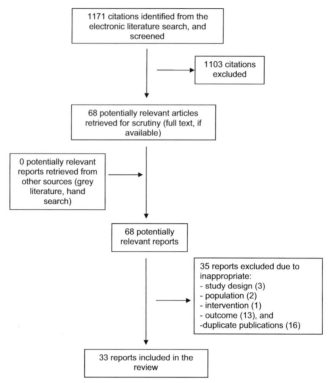

Fig. 1. Flow chart of selection of included studies for the review.

condition and, by far, are the most commonly used HRQL measures for clinical use. Dimensions captured by a specific measure are those most relevant to the area of key interest and may be more intuitive from a clinical perspective than generic measures. Because disease-specific measures center on those symptoms and disability specific to the condition they are more likely to be responsive to change than a generic health measure.[10,11] Unlike generic measures, the ability to make comparisons between different populations (eg, diseases) with specific measures of HRQL is limited.[12] In this review 16 studies[13–28] reviewed used the WOMAC and another 4 studies used the Oxford hip and knee scores[29–32] to evaluate joint-specific changes after total joint arthroplasty.

WOMAC Osteoarthritis Index
Seven studies of THA[13,16,17,21,25–27] **(Table 1)** and nine studies of TKA[14,15,18,19,20,22–24,28] **(Table 2)** assessed outcomes using the WOMAC Osteoarthritis Index. The WOMAC is a self-administered health questionnaire designed to measure disability of the osteoarthritic hip and knee.[33] It provides an aggregate score for each of the three subscales: joint pain (5 items), physical joint function (17 items), and joint stiffness (2 items).[33] Lower scores on the WOMAC dimensions reflect better health status (ie, less pain or stiffness and better function). A total score (ranging from 0 to 100) can also be calculated.[33]

The MCIDs for the domains of pain, functional limitations, and stiffness have been estimated to be 29, 27, and 26 points for THA, respectively.[26] These estimates were

Table 1
Disease-specific measures for total hip arthroplasty

Author, Year of Publication, Country	Study Design and Sample Size	Study Population	Measure/Domain	Baseline Mean (±SD) Score	Follow-up Mean (±SD) Score	Change	Effect Size
Fujita et al, 2009, Japan[17]	Prospective observational; n = 451	OA: 87.8%; Women: 84.5%; Age: 60.6 ± 10.0 years	WOMAC[a]	Approximately 2 days before surgery	6 weeks[a] / 6 months[a]	6 weeks[a] / 6 months[a]	6 weeks[a] / 6 months[a]
			Pain	39.5 ± 20.5	10.0 ± 11 / 7.5 ± 10.0	29.5 / 32.0	1.5 / 1.6
			Stiffness	35.0 ± 22.5	23.8 ± 15.0 / 17.5 ± 16.3	11.3 / 17.5	0.5 / 0.8
			Function	44.3 ± 20.3	21.9 ± 13.4 / 16.2 ± 12.2	22.4 / 28.1	1.1 / 1.4
Fielden et al, 2005, New Zealand[16]	Prospective observational; n = 122	OA; Women: 65%; Age: 66 (range, 35–85 years)	WOMAC	Within month before surgery	1 month / 3 months / 6 months	1 month / 3 months / 6 months	Unable to calculate
			Pain	54.5	28.5 / 12.5 / 8.5	4.0 / 24.5 / 30.0	
			Stiffness	75.0	36.2 / 22.5 / 17.5	5.0 / 31.2 / 43.8	
			Function	61.3	44.2 / 44.2 / 13.4	30.8 / 13.4 / 47.9	
Uesugi et al, 2009, Japan[32]	Prospective observational; n = 108	OA: 84.3%; Women: 79.6%; Age: 58.4 ± 12.5 years	OHS	2 days before surgery	6 months	6 months	6 months
			Global	32.6 ± 9.8	16.8 ± 6.6	15.8	1.6
			Pain	17.5 ± 5.5	8.3 ± 3.4	9.2	1.7
			Function	15.1 ± 5.1	8.6 ± 3.7	6.5	1.3
Clement et al, 2011, United Kingdom[29]	Prospective cohort	OA; Women: Older than 80: 63.7%, Control: 55.2%; Age: Older than 80 years n = 163, Older than 80–84.0 (range, 80–93 years); Control n = 376, Control: 70.3 (range, 65–74 years), Age: 65–74	OHS Global — Older than 80 years / Control	NR	NR	6 months / 1 year	Unable to calculate
			Global / Older than 80 years			19.8 / 19.8	
			Control			19.6 / 19.6	
			Pain / Older than 80 years			NR / 11.7 / 11.6	
			Control				
			Function / Older than 80 years			NR / 8.1 / 9.3	
			Control				

(continued on next page)

Table 1
(continued)

Author, Year of Publication, Country	Study Design and Sample Size	Study Population	Measure/Domain	Baseline Mean (±SD) Score	Follow-up Mean (±SD) Score	Change	Effect Size
Bachrach-Lindstrom et al, 2008, Sweden[13]	Prospective observational	OA Women: 48.9%	WOMAC[b]	Within 1 week before surgery	1 year	1 year	Unable to calculate
		Age Men: 69 ± 10 years Women: 70 ± 10 years	Pain Men	37 (30–45)	100 (95–100)	63	
			Women	35 (25–40)	100 (95–100)	65	
	n = 229 (men: 117; women: 112)		Stiffness Men	38 (25–50)	100 (75–100)	62	
			Women	25 (25–38)	88 (75–100)	63	
			Function Men	35 (29–42)	94 (88–98)	59	
			Women	32 (23–40)	91 (82–96)	59	
Ostendorf et al, 2004, Netherlands[25]	Prospective observational	OA: 83.3% Women: 62.3%	WOMAC[a]	NR	1 year	1 year	1 year
			Pain	58.5 ± 17.5	18.0 ± 21.5	40.5	2.3
		Age: 67.6 ± 10.1 years	Stiffness	61.3 ± 21.3	26.3 ± 21.3	35.0	1.7
	n = 114		Function	62.8 ± 16.8	22.9 ± 22.1	39.9	2.4
			OHS	42.5 ± 7.9	19.0 ± 7.7	23.5	3.0
SooHoo et al, 2007, United States[27]	Prospective observational	OA: NR Women: 54%	WOMAC	NR	17 months	17 months	17 months
		Age: 60 (range, 20–91) years	Global	51	19	32	1.5
	n = 89		Pain	10	3	8	1.5
			Stiffness	4	2	2	1.0
			Function	36	15	22	1.4

					While on waitlist	6 months	2 years	6 months	2 years	6 months	2 years
Quintana et al, 2005, Spain[26]	Prospective observational	OA: 100% Women: 50.7% Age: 69.4 ± 8.8 years	WOMAC	Pain	54.7 ± 18.7	15.1 ± 16.0	12.3 ± 17.3	39.6	42.4	2.1	2.2
	n = 469			Stiffness	58.0 ± 23.2	19.8 ± 18.6	15.5 ± 18.9	38.2	42.5	1.6	1.8
				Function	64.7 ± 16.3	26.7 ± 18.2	22.4 ± 19.4	38.1	42.4	2.3	2.6

					While on waitlist	1 year	7 years	1 year	7 years	1 year	7 years
Nilsdotter et al, 2010, Sweden[21]	Prospective observational	OA Women: 55% Age: 70 (range, 50–88) years	WOMAC	Pain	NR	85 ± 16.4	86 ±16.5	41	42	2.5	2.5
	n = 151			Stiffness	38 ± 15.9	77 ± 18.7	78 ± 22.1	39	40	2.5	2.5
				Function	38 ± 14.8	79 ± 16.7	76± 21.1	41	38	2.8	2.6

Abbreviations: NR, not reported; OHS, Oxford Hip Scale; OA, osteoarthritis; WOMAC, Western Ontario and McMaster Universities (WOMAC) Osteoarthritis Index.

a Transformed to a scale from 0 to 100 with lower scores reflective of less pain, stiffness, or dysfunction.

b Median (Q1–Q3).

Table 2
Disease-specific measures of total knee arthroplasty

Author, Year of Publication, Country	Study Design and Sample Size	Study Population	Measure/Domain	Baseline Mean (±SD) Score	Follow-up Mean (±SD) Score	Change	Effect Size
McQueen et al, 2007, United States[20]	Prospective observational n = 50	Women: 72% Age: 68 years (range, 54–80 years)	WOMAC Global Pain Stiffness Function	NR 47.1 9.7 3.4 33.5	6 months 79.4 17.2 5.5 56.7	6 months 32.3 7.4 2.1 22.8	Unable to calculate
Escobar et al, 2007, Spain[14]	Prospective observational n = 423	OA Women: 75% Age: 71.6 ± 6.7 years	WOMAC Pain Stiffness Function	NR 55.6 ± 18.5 61.9 ± 17.8 58.2 ± 24.1	6 months 31.6 ± 21.7 28.3 ± 21.6 27.2 ± 30.3	6 months 24.0 33.6 31.0	6 months 1.3 1.9 1.3
Escobar et al, 2007, Spain[15]	Prospective observational n = 640	OA Women: 74% Age: 71.8 ± 6.7 years	WOMAC Pain Stiffness Function	Completed while on waiting list 54.6 ± 18.2 56.1 ± 24.5 60.3 ± 17.7	6 months 22.9 ± 18.5 30.0 ± 22.5 32.1 ± 19.7	6 months 31.7 26.1 28.2	6 months 1.7 1.1 1.6
Jones et al, 2003, Canada[18]	Prospective observational n = 276	OA: 94% Women: 59% Age: 69.2 ± 9.2 years	WOMAC[a] Pain Stiffness Function	within 1 month before surgery 43.4 ± 17.4 39.7 ± 17.6 42.8 ± 21.5	6 months 76.0 ± 19.1 63.3 ± 22.0 70.5 ± 18.2	6 months 32.6 23.6 27.7	6 months 1.9 1.3 1.3

Study	Design	Population	n	Demographics	Instrument	Subscale								
							3 months before surgery	3 months	12 months		3 months	12 months		Unable to calculate
March et al, 2008, Australia[34]	Prospective observational	RA: 100% Women: 77%	n = 31	Age: 60.0 ± 14.9 years	HAQ		1.63	1.37	1.49		0.26	0.14		
							NR	**1 year**	**1 year**		**1 year**			**1 year**
Nunez et al, 2011, Spain[24]	Matched case control	Cases Women: 88% Age: 70.2 ± 6.7 years BMI: 39.9 ± 3.8 kg/m²	n = 63 cases (obese)		WOMAC	Pain Cases	58.6 ± 19.0	30.4 ± 20.4	36.0 (95% CI: 28.9–43.1)					1.9
						Control	55.0 ± 14.2	24.2 ± 18.9	30.8 (95% CI: 25.2–36.4)					2.2
						Stiffness Cases	53.3 ± 27.3	24.6 ± 22.5	28.7 (95% CI: 20.9–36.5)					1.1
						Control	37.9 ± 28.2	28.2 ± 26.5	9.7 (95% CI: 0.9–20.2)					0.3
		Controls Women: 88% Age: 71.7 years BMI: 29.4 ± 3.2 kg/m²	n = 63 controls (nonobese)			Function Cases	63.2 ± 17.2	22.6 ± 23.4	32.8 (95% CI: 38.8–26.8)					1.9
						Control	61.5 ± 14.5	30.0 ± 17.1	31.5 (5% CI: 36.9–26.2)					2.2
						Global Cases	61.4 ± 16.7	28.3 ± 20.0	33.1 (95% CI: 27.2–39.1)					2.0
						Control	58.2 ± 13.4	28.6 ± 17.1	29.6 (95% CI: 24.2–34.9)					2.2
							NR	**3 months**	**1 year**		**3 months**	**1 year**		**3 months 1 year**
Kirshner et al, 2003, Germany[19]	Prospective observational	OA Women: 76% Age: 71 (range, 58–86 years)	n = 63		WOMAC[b]	Global	NR	5.8 ± 2.6	2.9 ± 2.6		2.3	2.9		0.9 1.1
						Pain	5.6 ± 2.7	3.1 ± 2.8	2.5 ± 2.4	2.5	3.1		1.0 1.2	
						Stiffness	6.2 ± 3.2	4.0 ± 3.4	3.3 ± 3.1	2.2	2.9		0.7 0.9	
						Function	5.8 ± 2.8	3.5 ± 2.8	3.2 ± 2.8	2.3	2.6		0.8 0.9	
							NR	**3 months**	**6 months**	**12 months**	**3 months**	**6 months**	**12 months**	**3 months 6 months 12 months**
Terwee et al, 2006, Netherlands[28]	Prospective cohort	OA: NR Women: 77% Age: 68.7 ± 10.3 years	n = 163		WOMAC[a]	Pain	NR	46.9 ± 18.9	72.3 ± 19.1	77.6 ± 18.4	76.8 ± 19.9	25.4	30.7	29.9 1.3 1.6 1.6
						Function	45.2 + 18.8	67.2 + 21.0	72.1 + 18.7	71.7 ± 21.4	22.0	26.9	26.5 1.2 1.4 1.4

(continued on next page)

Table 2 (continued)

Author, Year of Publication, Country	Study Design and Sample Size	Study Population	Measure/Domain	Baseline Mean (±SD) Score	Follow-up Mean (±SD) Score	Change		Effect Size	
Clement et al, 2011, United Kingdom[29]	Prospective cohort	OA	OKS	NR	NR	6 months	1 year	Unable to calculate	
	Older than 80 years	Women: Older than 80 years: 63.2%	Global						
	n = 163	Controls: 55.1%	Older than 80 years			14.0	14.7		
			Control			14.2	15.8		
	Control	Age:	Pain						
	n = 435	Older than 80–83.3 years	Older than 80 years			NR	7.3		
	Age: 65–74	(range, 80–92 years)	Control				7.7		
		Control: 70.7 (range, 65–74 years)	Function						
			Older than 80 years			NR	7.4		
			Control				8.0		
Ko et al, 2011, Singapore[30]	Prospective observational	OA: NR Women: 79.5% Age: 67.1 ± 7.6 years	OKS	Several days before surgery	6 months	6 months	2 years	6 months	2 years
	n = 1716			36.6 ± 8.0	21.2 ± 6.5	15.4	17.6	1.9	2.2
Xie et al, 2010, Singapore[31]	Prospective observational	OA Women: 80.4%	OKS	One week before surgery	6 months	6 months	2 years	6 months	2 years
	n = 298	Age: 66.8 ± 7.6 years		49.1 ± 16.9	77.7 ± 15.4	28.6	34.0	1.7	2.0

(Ko et al Follow-up 2 years: 19.0 + 5.9; 83.1 ± 13.5 for Xie et al 2 years follow-up)

Study	Design	Population	n	Measure	Subscale	Baseline	Follow-up	Follow-up	Follow-up
Nunez et al, 2007, Spain[23]	Prospective observational	OA Women: 81% Age: 74.8 ± 5.6 years	n = 67	WOMAC		NR	3 years	3 years	3 years
					Pain	50.6 ± 12.7	23.2 ± 17.6	27.4 (95% CI: 21.7–33.1)	2.1
					Stiffness	31.8 ± 23.3	18.9 ± 20.3	13.0 (95% CI: 3.9–22.0)	0.6
					Function	54.3 ± 16.3	34.6 ± 17.9	19.7 (95% CI: 13.5–25.9)	1.2
Nunez et al, 2009, Spain[22]	Prospective observational	OA Women: 76.8% Age: 67.3 ± 16.6 years	n = 112	WOMAC		Day before surgery	7 years	7 years	7 years
					Global	54.2 ± 16.0	33.3 ± 21.3	20.9 (95% CI: 15.7–26.0)	1.3
					Pain	52.9 ± 16.3	25.9 ± 21.5	19.5 (95% CI: 14.0–24.9)	1.7
					Stiffness	43.3 ± 26.6	25.9 ± 25.5	17.4 (95% CI: 10.4–24.4)	0.7
					Function	55.8 ± 17.6	36.4 ± 22.7	20.9 (95% CI: 15.7–26.0)	1.1

†Abbreviations: BMI, body mass index; HAQ, Health Assessment Questionnaire; NR, not reported; OA, osteoarthritis; OKS, Oxford Knee Scale; RA, rheumatoid arthritis; WOMAC, Western Ontario and McMaster Universities (WOMAC) Osteoarthritis Index.

a Scoring reversed; higher scores are reflective of better outcome.

b Scores based on a 10-point scale with higher scores reflective of greater pain, stiffness, or dysfunction.

based on 379 patients who were recruited from three hospitals within a Spanish county from March 1999 to March 2000. Within the same setting, MCIDs for TKA were derived from 423 patients and were estimated to be 23, 19, and 15 points for pain, functional limitations, and stiffness, respectively.[14]

The Oxford Hip and Knee Scores

The Oxford Hip and Oxford Knee Scores assess outcomes of THA and TKA, respectively.[34] They are specific measures of HRQL that focus on the joint, excluding the impact of comorbidities when quantifying HRQL to improve responsiveness to an intervention such as THA or TKA. The scale consists of 12 items that assess pain and disability over the previous four weeks, related to the joint that is being evaluated. In the original scoring algorithm, each question has five response options and is scored on a 1- to 5-point scale, with lower scores indicating better function. An overall score is computed by summing the individual questions, creating a range of 12 (best) to 60 points (worse). An alternate scoring system assigns a value of 0 to 4 to each question, creating a range of 0 (worst) to 48 (best) for the overall score. The MCID of the Oxford Hip and Oxford Knee score has been estimated to be 3 to 5 points.[34]

Disease-Specific Outcomes

Total hip arthroplasty

Short-term outcomes Four studies assessed short-term outcomes within 6 months after THA (see **Table 1**).[16,17,26,32] In two studies, clinically important improvements were observed for all three WOMAC domains (approximately 30–48 points) 6 months after surgery.[16,26] In a 6-month observational study of 451 patients after THA, clinically important improvements were observed in the pain and function domains, but not stiffness.[17] Effect sizes (ES) were considered large, with the exception of the stiffness domain (ES = 0.5).[17]

Two studies[29,32] using the Oxford Hip Score (OHS) at 6 months after surgery found clinically important improvements, ranging from 6.5 to 15.8 points[32] for individual domains and approximately 20 points for global scores (see **Table 1**).[29]

Long-term outcomes Results reported after 1 year of follow-up were similar to those reported after 6 months. One study presented data for males and females separately and found clinically important improvements pain, stiffness and function for both genders of similar magnitude (59–65 points).[13] Similarly, two observational studies[21,25] reported clinically important changes in all three subscales of the WOMAC 1 year after THA (pain: 40.5–41 points; stiffness: 35.0–40 points and function: 38–39.9 points). Longer-term outcomes at 17 months,[27] 2 years,[26] and 7 years[21] demonstrated sustained improvements in WOMAC over baseline and large effect sizes in all subscales (ES =1.0–2.6).

One-year outcomes demonstrated clinically important changes in global OHS remain above the threshold of clinical important, but were smaller than those observed at 6 months (approximately 8–12 points over baseline) (see **Table 1**).[29] Although the effect sizes could not be calculated, another cohort study reported large effect sizes (ES = 3.0) at 1 year.[25]

Total knee arthroplasty

Short-term outcomes Clinically important improvements were seen with TKA in four[14,15,18,28] of five studies that assessed outcomes at 6 months after surgery for the pain, stiffness, and/or function subscales (see **Table 2**). Corresponding effect sizes were large, ranging from 1.1 to 1.9. An observational study of 50 patients reported clinically important change in function (22.8 points), although no variance was reported to estimate the effect size.[20]

As with the WOMAC, clinically important differences were reported with three studies [29,30,31] that used the Oxford Knee Score (OKS) at 6 months after surgery. Clinically important differences ranged from 14.0 to 28.6 points overall, with large corresponding effect sizes (ES = 1.7–1.9) (see **Table 2**).

Long-term outcomes Scores for the WOMAC at 1 year after TKA demonstrated clinically important improvements in the three WOMAC domains for 60 obese patients (body mass index [BMI] grades II, 35.0–39.9 kg/m^2 and III ≥40.0 kg/m^2): 36.0 (95% confidence interval [CI] 28.9, 43.1: pain), 28.7 (95% CI 20.9, 36.5: stiffness), and 32.8 (95% CI 26.8, 38.8: function) points. Clinically important changes were also reported for the 60 matched nonobese control participants for pain and function but not stiffness (9.7, 95% CI 0.9, 20.1 points). Effect sizes in cases and controls were large (ES = 1.1–2.2) for pain and function subscales.[24] Similar change and effect sizes were observed in another study that assessed the pain (change of 29.9 units) and function domains (change of 26.5 units).[28] These large changes were also seen at 36 months, which exceeded the threshold for clinical importance for the pain (27.4, 95% CI 21.7, 33.1 points; ES = 2.1) and function (19.7, 95% CI 13.5, 25.9 points; ES = 1.2) subscales, but not for the stiffness domain (13.0, 95% CI 3.9, 22.0 points), for which a moderate effect was observed (ES = 0.6).[23] A prospective 7-year cohort study of 112 patients reported improvement in pain that did not exceed the threshold of clinical importance (26.9, 95% CI 21.8, 32.1 points) yet the effect size was large (ES = 1.7).[22]

Long-term outcomes using the OKS at 1[29] to 2 years[30,31] also had clinically important differences (see **Table 2**).

The Health Assessment Questionnaire

Although the majority of studies examined joint arthroplasty in patients with osteoarthritis (OA), a 1-year observational study of 31 patients with rheumatoid arthritis (RA) examined pain and disability using the Health Assessment Questionnaire (HAQ).[35] The HAQ is a comprehensive measure for patients with a variety of rheumatic diseases, including RA. The Disability Index includes the ability to complete tasks such as dressing and grooming, rising, eating, walking, personal hygiene, reach, grip, and other activities.[36] Twenty items are used to assess the eight categories of functional activities. Scores on each dimension can be computed and then averaged to produce an overall score that ranges from 0.0 (best possible function) to 3.0 (worst function). The MCID on the HAQ is approximately 0.22 for persons with RA, but may be as low as 0.10 units.[36] At 3 months and 12 months after surgery, HAQ scores demonstrated clinically important improvements of 0.26 and 0.14 units, respectively.[35] Effect sizes could not be calculated for this study because the variances were not provided.

Generic Health Profiles

Generic measures of HRQL attempt to capture important aspects or dimensions of HRQL and are applicable across a broad range of conditions and populations. However, the broadness of generic HRQL measures can make them less responsive to changes in health status than specific measures. Because generic measures are multidimensional, they may lack the sensitivity of some areas of interest and have lower responsiveness than specific measures. A well-validated generic health measure will, however, permit the detection of unanticipated effects. Generic measures also provide for comparisons across different conditions, which have implications for health resource utilization and policy decisions. Within the total joint arthroplasty studies included in this scoping review, the SF-36 Health Survey (SF-36), SF-12 Health Survey (SF-12), Nottingham Profile (NHP), and the Sickness Impact Profile (SIP) were reported.

SF-36 and SF-12 health surveys
The SF-36 is a multidimensional generic health measure that examines eight health dimensions: physical function, role limitation (physical), bodily pain, mental health, emotional role function, social functioning, vitality, and general health perception.[37] Scoring for each dimension ranges from 0 to 100, with higher scores representing better health. There is no global score; however, two component summary measures, the physical component summary (PCS) and the mental component summary (MCS), have been derived from the eight dimensions and standardized using norm-based methods.[37] The summary scores describe the overall changes in HRQL, but may not capture the smaller changes within the specific dimensions.

The SF-12, which is a subset of the SF-36, includes two questions from the physical functioning, role-physical, role-emotional, and mental health domains and one item from the pain, vitality, social functioning, and general health dimensions of the SF-36. These 12 items are used to derive PCS-12 and MCS-12 scores, which are very similar to the physical and mental composite scores that would have been obtained using all items of the SF-36. The advantage of the SF-12 is its brevity, although complete data are required to derive the summary scores.[38]

In patients who underwent TKA, the MCID on the SF-36 ranged from 0.85 (general health) to 16.86 points (bodily pain).[14] For physical functioning, role physical, and social functioning, MCIDs were estimated to be 12 points, while the MCIDs for role emotional and vitality were smaller (8 and 4 points, respectively).[14] MCIDs ranged from 0.40 (general health) to 20 points (physical functioning) for THA.[26] The MCID for bodily pain was 15 points, role physical was 11 points, vitality was 10 points, and social functioning and general health were 9 points.[26] MCID for the PCS and MCS in patients with OA have been estimated to be approximately 4 and 2 points, respectively.[39] More generally, 5-point differences on the component scores have been considered clinically important.[40]

Nottingham Health Profile
The Nottingham Health Profile (NHP) assesses 6 dimensions of health using 38 questions with dichotomous yes/no response options: pain (5 items), physical mobility (8 items), emotional reactions (9 items), energy (3 items), social isolation (5 items), and sleep (5 items). Each of the six dimensions of the NHP is scored 0 (no problems at all for the dimension) to 100 (all problems for the dimension). Higher scores indicate greater dysfunction for a dimension.[41] One study found the clinically important differences for each domain to be: 35 points for pain, 29 points for physical mobility, 26 points for emotional reactions, 44 points for energy, 27 points for social isolation, and 18 points for sleep[42]; however, these values were not specific to orthopaedic patients.

Sickness Impact Profile
The Sickness Impact Profile (SIP) uses 136 items to assess 12 dimensions of health, including alertness behavior (10 items), ambulation (12 items), body care and movement (23 items), communication (9 items), eating (9 items), emotional behavior (9 items), home management (10 items), mobility (10 items), recreation and pastimes

(8 items), sleep and rest (7 items), social interaction (20 items), and work (9 items).[43] In addition, two overall domain scores (physical and psychosocial) or a single overall score can be computed. Scores on the SIP range from 0 to 100 for each individual domain, overall domain, or overall index, in which higher scores reflect worse health. Clinically important improvements on the physical functioning domain have been reported to be greater than 12.5 points and greater than 16 points on the psychosocial domain, but these values are not specific to orthopaedic surgery.[44]

Generic Outcomes

Total hip arthroplasty
Short-term outcomes As shown in **Table 3**, HRQL was evaluated with the SF-36 6 months after surgery in four studies.[26,32,45,46] Clinically important improvements were seen in all domains except bodily pain in an observational study of 335 patients using the Chinese version of the SF-36[45] and general health and mental health in 102 patients using the Polish version of the SF-36.[46] Large effect sizes were observed for the physical functioning, role-physical, and bodily pain domains.[26,32,46] Changes in the PCS and MCS were also clinically important in both studies, which reported summary scores.[45,46]

The magnitude of change measured with the SIP was 8.1 points at 3 months and 10.3 points at 6 months after THA, neither of which exceeded the threshold of clinical importance[47] (**Table 4**). Corresponding effect sizes were moderate at 3 months (ES = 0.5) and large at 6 months (ES = 0.8). Less change was seen for the psychosocial domain: 4.8 and 5.3 points after 3 and 6 months, respectively.

Long-term outcomes One year after THA, clinically important changes were reported in most SF-36 domains with the exception of general health,[21,25] bodily pain,[45] and mental health.[25] Effect sizes were large, ranging from 0.9 to 2.8 for most domains, but were moderate for the mental health domain (ES = 0.6) and small for the general health domain (ES = 0.3).[21] Three studies demonstrated clinically important improvements in the PCS scores 1 year[29,48] to 17 months[27] after THA (**Table 3**).

Longer-term outcomes, 2 to 7 years, demonstrated that postoperative gains in the physical functioning, role physical, general health, vitality, social functioning, and role emotional domains were maintained after 2 to 5 years,[45] while the physical functioning, role physical, bodily pain, and role emotional domains were maintained after 7 years.[21]

The NHP was used to assess the change in overall health 1 year after THA in prospective observational study of 229 patients (see **Table 4**).[13] Data for men (n = 117) and women (n = 112) were presented separately; however, the magnitude of the change was similar in both groups. For men and women, the change in mobility (42–43 points), pain (63–66 points), and sleep (31–36 points) were clinically important.

Total knee arthroplasty
Short-term outcomes Clinically important improvements and moderate to large effect sizes were observed for the SF-36 domains in seven studies (**Table 5**).[14,15,18,28,30,49,50] Two studies demonstrated smaller gains 6 months after TKA.[20,31]

Long-term outcomes Twelve-month data from a smaller observational study of patients with RA demonstrated clinically important changes in physical functioning, role physical, vitality, social functioning, and role emotional domains.[33] Participants with OA in larger studies reported clinically important improvements in physical

Table 3
SF-12 and SF-36 in total hip arthroplasty

Author, Year of Publication	Study Design and Sample Size	Study Population	Measure/ Domains	Baseline Mean (±SD) Score	Follow-up Mean (±SD) Score	Change	Effect Size
Uesugi et al, 2009, Japan[32]	Prospective observational n = 108	OA: 84.3% Women: 79.6% Age: 58.4 ± 12.5 years	SF-36	2 days before surgery	6 months	6 months	6 months
			PF	39.7 ± 21.7	71.9 ± 19.8	32.2	1.5
			RP	49.4 ± 30.1	78.5 ± 25.3	29.1	1.0
			BP	39.1 ± 19.4	73.1 ± 22.0	34.0	1.8
			GH	58.3 ± 19.7	63.8 ± 19.3	5.5	0.3
			VT	53.2 ± 21.7	67.8 ± 19.4	14.6	0.7
			SF	57.9 ± 28.7	82.4 ± 25.2	24.5	0.9
			RE	61.6 ± 31.7	84.4 ± 24.5	22.8	0.7
			MH	64.0 ± 22.2	75.0 ± 18.6	11.0	0.5
Badura-Brozoza et al, 2009, Poland[46]	Prospective observational n = 102	OA Women: 57.8% Median age: 61 years (range, 54–75) years	SF-36	Two weeks before surgery	6 months	6 months	6 months
			PF	28.9 ± 18.5	52.3 ± 27.1	23.4	1.3
			RP	15.4 ± 28.6	44.2 ± 40.3	28.8	1.0
			BP	20.1 ± 21.3	56.8 ± 26.5	36.7	1.7
			GH	48.1 ± 17.2	51.1 ± 19.9	3.0	0.2
			VT	48.8 ± 17.2	59.5 ± 17.2	10.7	0.6
			SF	52.5 ± 23.7	69.7 ± 26.3	17.2	0.7
			RE	40.1 ± 44.3	58.5 ± 44.7	18.4	0.4
			MH	59.1 ± 20.3	66.8 ± 18.1	7.7	0.4
			PCS	28.7 ± 5.8	42.9 ± 8.6	14.2	2.4
			MCS	47.1 ± 10.4	53.1 ± 12.4	6.0	0.6

Study	Study design / sample	Population	SF-12	Within 6 weeks of surgery / NR	1 year	1 year	Unable to calculate
Clement et al, 2011, United Kingdom[29]	Prospective cohort; Over 80 years; n = 163; Control age 65 to 74 years; n = 376	OA Women: Older than 80 years: 63.7%; Control: 55.2%; Age: Older than 80 years: 84.0 (range, 80–93) years; Control: 70.3 (range, 65–74) years	PCS — over 80 years	NR	NR		Unable to calculate
			PCS — Control			10.3	
			MCS — Older than 80 years			14.4	
			MCS — Control			1.8	
						3.1	
Dowsey et al, 2010, Australia[48]	Prospective cohort; n = 471; BMI nonobese: n = 277; obese: n = 173; morbidly obese n = 21	OA: 84%; Women: 60.7%; Age: 68.9 ± 10.4 years; BMI	PCS — Nonobese	25.7 ± 5.6	40.0 ± 11.4	14.3 ± 11.2	2.6
			PCS — Obese	25.3 ± 4.5	37.5 ± 11.0	12.2 ± 11.8	2.7
			PCS — Morbidly obese	22.9 ± 3.6	33.6 ± 10.2	10.7 ± 10.3	3.0
			MCS — Nonobese	50.8 ± 9.8	50.7 ± 11.8	−0.1 ± 11.7	0.0
			MCS — Obese	46.9 ± 10.4	50.8 ± 10.5	3.6 ± 12.2	0.3
			MCS — Morbidly obese	47.2 ± 10.3	50.9 ± 9.7	3.7 ± 9.4	0.4

(continued on next page)

Table 3
(continued)

Author, Year of Publication	Study Design and Sample Size	Study Population	Measure/ Domains	Baseline Mean (±SD) Score	Follow-up Mean (±SD) Score	Change	Effect Size
Ostendorf et al, 2004, Netherlands[25]	Prospective observational n = 114	OA: 83.3% Women: 62.3% Age: 67.6 ± 10.1 years	SF-36	NR	1 year	1 year	1 year
			PF	22.0 ± 16.9	60.7 ± 26.0	38.7	2.3
			RP	11.0 ± 24.0	55.3 ± 47.1	44.3	1.9
			BP	28.5 ± 16.5	72.1 ± 26.3	43.6	2.6
			GH	63.8 ± 19.8	66.7 ± 20.4	2.9	0.1
			VT	55.1 ± 21.3	68.4 ± 21.0	13.3	0.6
			SF	55.7 ± 29.7	79.2 ± 25.7	23.5	0.8
			RE	51.7 ± 43.5	68.7 ± 43.0	17.0	0.4
			MH	73.5 ± 19.4	79.4 ± 19.8	5.9	0.3
			SF-12				
			PCS	30.5 ± 8.3	45.6 ± 9.6	15.1	1.8
			MCS	41.4 ± 12.5	49.7 ± 12.2	8.3	0.7
SooHoo et al, 2007, United States[27]	Prospective observational n = 89	OA: NR Women: 54% Age: 60 (range, 20–91 years)	SF-36	NR	17 months	17 months	17 months
			PF	23	61	37	2.0
			RP	24	58	34	0.9
			BP	30	61	31	1.5
			GH	66	61	−6	−0.2
			VT	49	60	11	0.5
			SF	58	77	20	0.7
			RE	56	74	18	0.4
			MH	67	76	9	0.4
			PCS	31	42	12	1.5
			MCS	50	52	2	0.2

Quintana et al, 2005, Spain[26] — Prospective observational; OA; Women: 50.7%; Age: 69.4 ± 8.8 years; n = 469; SF-36

	While on waitlist	6 months	2 years	6 months	2 years	6 months	2 years
PF	21.5 ± 20.7	54.5 ± 25.0	56.3 ± 28.0	33.0	34.8	1.6	1.7
RP	11.0 ± 27.3	44.1 ± 44.6	59.5 ± 43.7	33.1	48.6	1.2	1.8
BP	31.0 ± 26.0	61.5 ± 29.4	64.7 ± 29.7	30.5	33.7	1.2	1.3
GH	58.7 ± 19.6	63.9 ± 20.0	61.7 ± 22.2	5.3	3.0	0.3	0.2
VT	42.7 ± 23.6	62.3 ± 24.0	62.5 ± 25.3	19.7	19.8	0.8	0.8
SF	55.2 ± 31.6	78.9 ± 24.7	79.4 ± 24.7	23.8	24.2	0.8	0.8
RE	67.0 ± 44.7	82.1 ± 37.0	82.1 ± 35.8	15.2	15.1	0.3	0.3
MH	60.0 ± 23.3	73.5 ± 22.3	73.4 ± 22.4	13.6	13.4	0.6	0.6

Shi et al, 2009, Taiwan[45] — Prospective observational; OA; Women: 43.3%; Age: 59.8 ± 14.7 years; n = 335; SF-36[a]

	While on waitlist	Preoperative	3 months	6 months	1 year	2 years	5 years	3 months	6 months	1 year	2 years	5 years	Effect size
PF	NR	39.8 ± 3.9	60.4 ± 1.9	69.6 ± 1.9	78.7 ± 2.0	80.9 ± 2.3	87.9 ± 1.8	20.6	29.8	38.9	41.1	48.1	Unable to calculate
RP	NR	12.2 ± 5.9	39.3 ± 2.9	48.4 ± 3.1	64.5 ± 3.2	78.0 ± 3.2	90.3 ± 2.5	27.1	36.2	52.3	65.8	78.1	
BP	NR	42.3 ± 1.3	47.9 ± 0.8	48.4 ± 0.7	49.3 ± 0.8	49.5 ± 0.7	49.8 ± 0.6	5.6	6.1	7.0	7.2	7.5	
GH	NR	52.0 ± 3.2	61.7 ± 1.6	64.0 ± 1.7	66.8 ± 1.7	69.4 ± 1.8	79.9 ± 1.6	9.7	12.0	14.8	17.4	27.9	
VT	NR	56.2 ± 3.3	66.9 ± 1.4	67.7 ± 1.5	70.8 ± 1.5	71.4 ± 1.8	82.9 ± 1.7	10.7	11.5	14.6	15.2	26.7	
SF	NR	60.9 ± 3.8	66.6 ± 1.6	74.9 ± 1.6	81.5 ± 1.7	88.7 ± 1.9	95.0 ± 1.7	5.7	14.0	20.6	27.8	34.1	
RE	NR	43.6 ± 6.1	77.4 ± 3.3	85.7 ± 3.4	88.3 ± 3.3	90.0 ± 3.5	95.1 ± 3.2	33.8	42.1	44.7	46.4	51.5	
MH	NR	62.0 ± 2.7	71.5 ± 1.2	72.6 ± 1.2	73.0 ± 1.3	74.4 ± 1.6	83.1 ± 1.6	9.5	10.6	10.9	12.4	21.1	
PCS	NR	25.8 ± 1.5	30.4 ± 0.8	33.6 ± 0.8	37.7 ± 0.8	39.9 ± 0.8	43.3 ± 0.6	4.7	7.9	11.9	14.1	17.5	
MCS	NR	47.7 ± 1.5	54.0 ± 0.8	55.0 ± 0.8	55.4 ± 0.8	56.0 ± 0.9	59.9 ± 0.9	6.3	7.3	7.7	8.3	12.2	

Nilsdotter et al, 2010, Sweden[21] — Prospective observational; OA; Women: 55%; Age: 70 (range, 50–88 years); n = 151; SF-36

	While on waitlist	Preoperative	1 year	7 years	1 year	7 years	1 year	7 years
PF	NR	31 ± 19.4	68 ± 21.1	54 ± 27.2	37	23	1.9	1.2
RP	NR	9 ± 21.1	61 ± 41.2	45 ± 44.6	52	36	2.5	1.7
BP	NR	31 ± 15.8	75 ± 22.7	63 ± 28.1	44	32	2.8	2.0
GH	NR	68 ± 19.8	73 ± 21.6	63 ± 22.4	5	−5	0.3	0.3
VT	NR	49 ± 20.2	73 ± 20.6	59 ± 46.4	24	10	1.2	0.5
SF	NR	63 ± 26.4	88 ± 21.3	62 ± 23.8	25	−1	0.9	0.0
RE	NR	37 ± 43.5	74 ± 36.8	81 ± 23.2	37	44	0.9	1.0
MH	NR	70 ± 21.1	83 ± 18.9	79 ± 19.1	13	9	0.6	0.4

Abbreviations: NR, not reported; OA, osteoarthritis; PF, physical function; RP, physical role limitation; BP, bodily pain; GH, general health; VT, vitality; SF, social function; RE, emotional role limitation; MH, mental health; PCS, physical component summary; MCS, mental component summary.

[a] Standard error reported.

Table 4
Other generic health profiles in total hip arthroplasty

Author, Year of Publication, Country	Study Design and Sample Size	Study Population	Measure/Domain	Baseline Mean (±SD) Score	Follow-up Mean (±SD) Score		Change		Effect Size	
					3 months	6 months	3 months	6 months	3 months	6 months
Montin et al, 2011, Finland[47]	Prospective observational	OA	SIP	The day before surgery						
	n = 100	Women: 54%	Total	13.4 ± 9.7	7.2 ± 8.5	6.0 ± 7.7	6.2	7.4	0.6	0.8
		Age: 63.9 ± 11.6 years	Physical	16.6 ± 13.1	8.5 ± 11.5	6.3 ± 10.0	8.1	10.3	0.5	0.8
			Psychosocial	9.2 ± 9.8	4.4 ± 6.8	3.9 ± 6.2	4.8	5.3	0.5	0.5
Bachrach-Lindstrom et al, 2008, Sweden[13]	Prospective observational	OA	NHP[a]	Within 1 week before surgery	1 year		1 year		Unable to calculate	
	n = 229	Women: 48.9%	Mobility							
	(men: 117; women: 112)	Age:	Men	53 (38–68)	10 (0–16)		43			
		Men: 69 ± 10.0 years	Women	53 (46–68)	11 (0–28)		42			
		Women: 70 ± 10.0 years	Pain							
			Men	63 (46–82)	0 (0–0)		63			
			Women	66 (53–88)	0 (0–8)		66			
			Sleep							
			Men	31 (11–53)	0 (0–11)		31			
			Women	36 (20–62)	0 (0–23)		36			
			Energy							
			Men	39 (0–63)	0 (0–5)		39			
			Women	41 (24–63)	0 (0–11)		41			
			Social Isolation							
			Men	0 (0–7)	0 (0–0)		0			
			Women	0 (0–7)	0 (0–0)		0			
			Emotional reactions							
			Men	8 (0–13)	0 (0–0)		8			
			Women	8 (0–22)	0 (0–7)		8			
			Total score							
			Men	33 (23–42)	3 (0–9)		30			
			Women	36 (30–48)	7 (2–12)		29			

Abbreviations: NHP, Nottingham Health Profile; OA, osteoarthritis; SIP, sickness impact profile.

a Median (Q1–Q3).

functioning scores over 1 and 2 years.[28,30,31] Although large effect sizes were found with bodily pain in many studies,[19,28,30] no change in bodily pain was seen in one large study of Chinese participants in spite of reported large effect sizes with the OKS.[31]

The SF-12 was used to assess 1-year outcomes after THA and TKA in 185 patients who were 80 years or older compared to 492 patients 65 to 74 years[29] (see **Tables 3** and **5**). Twelve months after THA, gains in the PCS were clinically important (10.3 points for those older than age 80 years and 14.4 points in the control group). Similarly, larger gains were seen with the PCS in younger patients (10.6 points) compared to older (7.9 points) (see **Table 5**). Changes in the MCS were minimal for both groups.

Preference-Based Measures

Generic HRQL measures can be further categorized as health profiles and index measures. Health profiles provide separate scores for each dimension or domain, whereas index measures provide an overall summary score. Utility measures are one type of index measure and were developed from economics and decision theory. A preference-based measure places an overall value on a health state that is useful in both the clinical and health policy settings. Valuations of heath states, however, are dependent on the measure and may account for differences in scores across measures.[51] Patients' preferences are front and foremost in clinical care, and providing a value to these preferences can provide important information for both clinicians and patients. Health policy requires comparison across conditions to evaluate the treatment effect and economic implications of interventions and/or programs.[52]

An assumption of HRQL is that individuals have preferences for alternative health outcomes. Scores are anchored on a scale in which dead = 0.00 and perfect health = 1.00. Negative scores are also possible and reflect health states that are considered worse than dead. From an economic perspective, a preference-based measure may be useful to assess HRQL. There are several advantages of a utility measure. First, the single summary score provides the ability to deal with any conflicting changes in various dimensions of health states, for instance, an improvement in function accompanied by a dramatic increase in pain. On the other hand, many of the scales do not cover the same aspects of health. For example, the Quality of Well-Being (QWB) measures performance of an activity (eg, does a person climb stairs?), whereas others evaluate capacity (eg is a person able to climb stairs?). Second, a single index value can be generated for cost-effectiveness analyses. Mortality and morbidity effects can be integrated by estimating quality-adjusted life years (QALYs). Within the context of this review, EQ-5D, QWB, SF-6D, and 15-D were used to evaluate the effectiveness of total joint arthroplasty.

EQ-5D

The EQ-5D assesses five attributes of health (mobility, self-care, usual activities, pain, and anxiety/depression).[53] Patients are asked to think about their health "today" and characterize themselves as having no problems, moderate problems, or severe problems on each attribute. This creates a health status classification system, to which a multiattribute utility function is then applied to obtain an overall score. The lowest possible overall score (corresponding to severe problems on all five attributes) varies depending on the utility function that is applied to the health classification system (eg, -0.59 for the U.K. algorithm and -0.109 for the U.S. algorithm). Scores less than 0 represent health states that are valued by society as being worse than

Table 5
SF-12 and SF-36 in total knee arthroplasty

Author, Year of Publication, Country	Study Design and Sample Size	Study Population	Measure/Domain	Baseline Mean (±SD) Score	Follow-up Mean (±SD) Score 3 months	Follow-up Mean (±SD) Score 6 months	Change 3 months	Change 6 months	Effect Size 3 months	Effect Size 6 months
Tsonga et al, 2011, Greece[49]	Prospective, single group	OA Women: 100%	SF-36	One week before surgery	3 months	6 months	3 months	6 months	3 months	6 months
			PF	29.4 ± 12.4	64.1 ± 19.3	73.3 ± 22.8	34.8	44.0	2.8	3.5
	n = 52	Age: 72.6 ± 5.9 years	RP	0.98 ± 3.8	19.0 ± 29.7	28.8 ± 31.5	18.0	27.9	4.7	7.3
			BP	18.4 ± 9.6	65.1 ± 12.5	72.1 ± 15.1	46.7	53.7	4.9	5.6
			GH	46.1 ± 8.3	50.1 ± 6.7	52.5 ± 4.3	4.0	6.4	0.5	0.8
			VT	38.2 ± 12.4	63.3 ± 10.3	67.5 ± 8.0	25.1	29.2	2.0	2.4
			SF	45.7 ± 24.8	67.8 ± 25.8	76.4 ± 20.8	22.1	30.7	0.9	1.2
			RE	12.9 ± 19.4	45.2 ± 48.6	65.1 ± 44.0	32.3	52.1	1.7	2.7
			MH	43.0 ± 15.3	66.1 ± 12.3	63.1 ± 9.1	23.2	20.2	1.5	1.3
			PCS	23.7 ± 1.9	49.6 ± 2.6	56.7 ± 2.9	26.4	33.0	13.9	17.4
			MSC	35.0 ± 2.9	60.7 ± 20.8	68.0 ± 15.3	25.8	33.0	8.9	11.4
Peterlein et al, 2009, Germany[50]	Prospective observational	OA Women: 69.2%	SF-36	NR	6 months		6 months		6 months	
			PF	21.1 ± 12.1	54.3 ± 25.2		33.2		2.7	
	n = 52	Age: 68.1 ± 9.1 years	RP	12.5 ± 27.8	40.5 ± 41.0		28.0		1.0	
			BP	16.1 ± 12.8	52.6 ± 28.2		36.5		2.9	
			GH	NR	NR		Unable to calculate		Unable to calculate	
			VT	42.4 ± 21.4	56.2 ± 21.2		13.8		0.6	
			SF	51.8 ± 31.3	78.6 ± 27.5		26.8		0.9	
			RE	41.7 ± 49.3	72.6 ± 43.0		30.9		0.6	
			MH	NR	NR		Unable to calculate		Unable to calculate	

Study	Design		Demographics		Instrument	Subscale	NR	6 months	6 months	6 months
McQueen et al, 2007, United States[20]	Prospective observational	OA	Women: 72% Age: 68 years (range, 54–80 years)	n = 50	SF-36	PF	14.3	20.1	5.8	Unable to calculate
						RP	4.7	6.3	1.6	
						BP	5.0	8.0	3.0	
						GH	18.2	18.3	0.2	
						VT	12.5	14.7	2.2	
						SF	6.8	8.7	1.9	
						RE	4.7	5.3	0.6	
						MH	18.3	19.2	0.9	
						PCS	24.2	34.6	10.4	
						MCS	30.0	33.2	3.2	
							NR	6 months	6 months	6 months
Escobar et al, 2007, Spain[14]	Prospective observational	OA	Women: 75% Age: 71.6 ± 6.7 years	n = 423	SF-36	PF	23.9 ± 21.2	Values NR	23.4 ± 28.2	1.1
						RP	14.0 ± 29.3		28.3 ± 46.0	0.5
						BP	34.7 ± 28.5		18.8 ± 33.7	1.2
						GH	57.8 ± 20.6		2.8 ± 18.6	2.8
						VT	43.3 ± 25.4		11.6 ± 25.1	1.8
						SF	56.0 ± 31.7		16.9 ± 33.7	1.4
						RE	63.5 ± 46.0		9.8 ± 50.1	1.7
						MH	59.3 ± 24.2		7.7 ± 23.5	2.5
							While on waitlist	6 months	6 months	6 months
Escobar et al, 2007, Spain[15]	Prospective observational	OA	Women: 74% Age: 71.8 ± 6.7 years	n = 640	SF-36	PF	25.0 ± 21.4	48.8 ± 24.2	23.8	1.1
						RP	17.0 ± 31.6	44.8 ± 43.8	27.8	0.9
						BP	36.5 ± 27.7	54.6 ± 30.0	18.1	0.7
						GH	58.6 ± 20.0	61.0 ± 21.0	2.4	0.1
						VT	44.8 ± 24.8	56.8 ± 24.7	12.0	0.5
						SF	58.7 ± 31.3	74.9 ± 27.3	16.2	0.5
						RE	66.4 ± 45.3	74.5 ± 41.0	8.1	0.2
						MH	60.2 ± 24.3	68.1 ± 23.9	7.9	0.3

(continued on next page)

Table 5
(continued)

Author, Year of Publication, Country	Study Design and Sample Size	Study Population	Measure/ Domain	Baseline Mean (±SD) Score	Follow-up Mean (±SD) Score	Change	Effect Size
Jones et al, 2003, Canada[18]	Prospective observational n = 276	OA: 94% Women: 59% Age: 69.2 ± 9.2 years	SF-36	NR	6 months	6 months	6 months
			PF	21.0 ± 18.1	44.8 ± 25.3	23.8	1.3
			RP	12.0 ± 24.7	35.2 ± 40.0	23.2	0.9
			BP	30.8 ± 17.6	53.4 ± 22.8	22.6	1.3
			GH	62.1 ± 19.4	64.5 ± 19.8	2.4	0.1
			VT	42.0 ± 20.9	52.9 ± 22.7	10.9	0.5
			SF	54.0 ± 27.2	72.1 ± 27.7	18.1	0.7
			RE	55.2 ± 44.3	67.3 ± 40.4	12.1	0.3
			MH	68.9 ± 19.5	75.0 ± 19.0	6.1	0.3
			PCS	25.9 ± 7.5	34.6 ± 10.1	8.7	1.2
			MCS	50.1 ± 11.4	52.5 ± 10.8	2.4	0.2
Tervee et al, 2006, Netherlands[28]	Prospective n = 163	OA: NR Women: 77% Age: 68.7 ± 10.3 years	SF-36	NR	3 months / 6 months / 12 months	3 months / 6 months / 12 months	3 months / 6 months / 12 months
			PF	29.2 ± 19.3	48.0 ± 22.5 / 55.9 ± 21.5 / 52.3 ± 22.7	18.8 / 26.7 / 23.1	1.0 / 1.4 / 1.2
			BP	35.2 ± 20.0	56.7 ± 23.3 / 66.1 ± 23.8 / 65.6 ± 24.7	21.5 / 30.9 / 30.4	1.1 / 1.5 / 1.5
March et al, 2008, Australia[34]	Prospective observational n = 31	RA Women: 77% Age: 60 ± 14.9 years	SF-36	3 months before surgery	3 months / 1 year	3 months / 1 year	Unable to calculate
			PF	26.6	38.5 / 40.6	11.9 / 14.0	
			RP	17.9	34.3 / 35.7	16.4 / 17.8	
			BP	34.7	45.2 / 48.8	10.5 / 14.1	
			GH	50.3	53.2 / 50.9	2.9 / 0.6	
			VT	44.1	46.1 / 49.2	2.0 / 5.1	
			SF	61.2	70.4 / 76.7	9.2 / 15.5	
			RE	63.1	53.8 / 76.2	−9.3 / 13.1	
			MH	60.4	70.8 / 73.5	10.4 / 13.1	
			PCS	27.8	32.2 / 31.1	4.4 / 3.3	
			MCS	48.4	49.9 / 54.1	1.5 / 5.7	

In the table below the three mean ± SD columns give the Preoperative, 3-month, and 1-year scores; the next pair of "3 months / 1 year" columns give the change from baseline; the final pair of "3 months / 1 year" columns give the standardized response mean (SRM).

Study	Design	Sample	Instrument	Subscale	Baseline	Preoperative (mean ± SD)	3 months (mean ± SD)	1 year (mean ± SD)	3 months (change)	1 year (change)	3 months (SRM)	1 year (SRM)
Kirshner et al, 2003, Germany[19]	Prospective observational	OA; Women: 76%; Age: 71 (range, 58–86 years); n = 63	SF-36	PF	NR	24.0 ± 20.3	36.0 ± 24.6	43.3 ± 28.1	12	19.3	0.6	1.0
				RP		15.7 ± 31.5	33.5 ± 40.7	45.1 ± 44.1	17.8	29.4	0.6	0.9
				BP		26.5 ± 18.9	50.2 ± 29.3	58.6 ± 29.0	23.7	32.1	1.3	1.7
				GH		55.0 ± 19.3	51.3 ± 18.3	54.4 ± 20.1	-3.7	-0.6	-0.2	-0.03
				VT		45.8 ± 19.6	53.0 ± 21.8	52.3 ± 21.5	7.2	6.5	0.4	0.3
				SF		68.2 ± 25.9	79.6 ± 23.8	81.0 ± 22.5	11.4	12.8	0.4	0.5
				RE		44.1 ± 45.7	58.0 ± 45.4	53.5 ± 46.0	13.9	9.4	0.3	0.2
				MH		61.6 ± 20.3	68.8 ± 20.3	68.2 ± 20.4	7.2	6.6	0.4	0.3
Clement et al, 2011, United Kingdom[29]	Prospective cohort	OA; Women: Older than 80: 63.2%, Control: 55.1%; n = 185 over the age of 80; Control: n = 492 age 65 to 74 (control group); Age: Older than 80: 80–84.0 years, Control: 70.7 years	SF-12	PCS — Older than 80 years	NR	NR	NR	NR		7.9		Unable to calculate
				PCS — Control	NR	NR	NR	NR		0.6		Unable to calculate
				MSC — Older than 80 years	NR	NR	NR	NR		10.6		Unable to calculate
				MSC — Control	NR	NR	NR	NR		-0.4		Unable to calculate

(continued on next page)

Table 5
(continued)

Author, Year of Publication, Country	Study Design and Sample Size	Study Population	Measure/ Domain	Baseline Mean (±SD) Score	Follow-up Mean (±SD) Score		Change		Effect Size	
					6 months	2 years	6 months	2 years	6 months	2 years
Xie et al, 2010, Singapore[31]	Prospective observational	OA Women: 80.4%	SF-36	1 week before surgery						
	n = 298	Age: 66.8 ± 7.6 years	PF	37.2 ± 20.2	55.4 ± 23.4	59.8 ± 23.6	22.5 ± 1.7	26.7 ± 2.1	1.1	1.3
			RP	38.8 ± 40.7	71.9 ± 41.5	68.9 ± 42.7	32.9 ± 3.4	28.7 ± 4.5	0.8	0.7
			BP	41.7 ± 14.3	47.6 ± 18.0	40.9 ± 14.0	6.0 ± 1.5	−0.57 ± 1.6	0.4	0.0
			GH	56.1 ± 8.9	56.2 ± 9.0	52.2 ± 8.3	0.12 ± 0.8	−4.1 ± 0.9	0.0	0.5
			VT	56.4 ± 12.8	56.2 ± 13.4	55.9 ± 11.2	−0.20 ± 0.9	−0.58 ± 1.3	0.0	0.0
			SF	52.8 ± 14.0	54.3 ± 15.6	51.0 ± 9.7	1.5 ± 1.3	−1.52 ± 1.2	0.1	0.1
			RE	81.2 ± 38.6	96.8 ± 16.2	93.3 ± 23.8	15.6 ± 2.6	12.2 ± 3.2	0.4	0.3
			MH	64.7 ± 10.2	65.9 ± 11.4	65.5 ± 8.7	1.2 ± 0.9	0.57 ± 1.0	0.1	0.1
Ko et al, 2011, Singapore[30]	Prospective observational	OA: NR Women: 79.5% Age: 67.1 ± 7.6 years	SF-36	several days before surgery						
	n = 1716		PF	33.1 ± 21.0	59.7 ± 21.8	65.2 ± 22.4	26.6	32.1	1.3	1.5
			RP	33.7 ± 42.1	74.0 ± 39.9	77.8 ± 38.3	40.3	44.1	1.0	1.0
			BP	38.0 ± 18.6	71.1 ± 23.9	73.9 ± 24.9	33.1	35.9	1.8	1.9
			GH	72.6 ± 20.0	74.5 ± 19.7	73.6 ± 20.7	1.9	1.0	0.1	0.1
			VT	64.5 ± 21.6	70.5 ± 19.7	72.0 ± 19.8	6.0	7.5	0.3	0.3
			SF	57.3 ± 35.3	84.6 ± 27.4	87.6 ± 26.9	27.3	30.3	0.8	0.9
			RE	77.6 ± 40.8	93.0 ± 24.6	93.0 ± 24.8	15.4	15.4	0.4	0.4
			MH	73.9 ± 20.0	80.5 ± 15.7	81.1 ± 16.9	6.6	7.2	0.3	0.4

Abbreviations: BP, bodily pain; GH, general health; MH, mental health; NR, not reported; OA, osteoarthritis; PCS, component summary; PF, physical function; RA, rheumatoid arthritis; RE, emotional role limitation; RP, physical role limitation; SF, social function; VT, vitality.

dead, while scores of 0 and 1.00 are assigned to the health states "dead" and "perfect health," respectively. The score obtained from the multiattribute utility function is often referred to as the EQ-5D scale score, index score or tariff. The EQ-5D also includes a visual analog scale (EQ-5D VAS). The scale is anchored with "worst imaginable health state" at the bottom and "best imaginable health state" at the top. Possible scores range along the scale range from 0 to 100. Estimates of the MCID for the EQ-5D utility score range from 0.01 to 0.14 and average 0.07 units.[53]

Quality of well-being

The QWB assesses three attributes of HRQL, including mobility (three levels), physical activity (three levels), and social activity (five levels).[53] In addition to the three attributes, the QWB includes an assessment of 21 symptoms and problems (referred to as symptom/problem complexes) experienced over the previous 8 days. Symptoms pertaining to emotional health, cognitive function, speech, general weakness, arm function, and eye function are assessed. The symptom/problem complexes are scored as present or absent and the most severe one contributes to the overall score. Scores on the QWB range from 0.0 (dead) to 1.0 (complete well-being), but the lowest possible score for a living person is 0.33. The QWB does not have negative scores (states worse than dead). The MCID for the QWB is estimated to be 0.03 units, although higher values have been observed in some conditions.[53]

SF-6D

The SF-6D is a utility measure based upon a selection of questions from the SF-36.[53] The SF-6D evaluates six attributes of HRQL including physical functioning, role limitations, social functioning, pain, mental health, and vitality. Each attribute of the SF-6D has four to six levels of functioning. Scores on the SF-6D range from 0.0 (dead) to 1.0 (perfect health), with the lowest possible score for a living person being 0.32. The SF-6D does not have negative scores (states worse than dead).[53] The SF-6D has floor effects when compared to other utility measures, particularly with functional activities. In knee and hip replacement, the MCIDs for the SF-6D was estimated to be 0.04[14] and 0.09[26], respectively.

15D

The 15D assesses 15 attributes of health (moving, seeing, hearing, breathing, sleeping, eating, speech, eliminating, usual activities, mental function, discomfort and symptoms, depression, distress, vitality, and sexual activity).[54,55] Respondents are asked to rate their present state on each dimension, selecting one of five levels that best describes themselves. The 15 dimensions can be used to create a generic health profile or to create an overall index score, through the application of a multiattribute utility function. The maximum score on the 15-D is 1 (no problems in any dimension) and the minimum score is 0 (dead). The 15-D does not have negative scores (states worse than dead). The MCID on the 15-D has been estimated to be 0.03 points,[55] although this value is not specific to joint replacement.

Outcomes Using Utility Measures

Total hip arthroplasty

Compared to baseline, clinically important changes in EQ-5D utility scores were reported over 1 year after surgery[13,16,17,25,56–58] (**Table 6**). The long-term effect sizes of the EQ-5D were large regardless of the timing of assessment, ranging from 1.0 to 1.8. A similar large effect size (ES = 1.1) was seen with the QWB score at 1 year (see **Table 6**).[59] Clinically important gains were seen at 6 months (0.16) and 2 years (0.18)

Table 6
Generic utility measures in total hip arthroplasty

Author, Year of Publication, Country	Study Design and Sample Size	Study Population	Measure/Domain	Baseline Mean (±SD) Score	Follow-up Mean (±SD) Score	Change	Effect Size
Fujita et al, 2009, Japan[17]	Prospective observational; n = 451	OA: 87.8%, Women: 84.5%, Age: 60.6 ± 10.0 years		Approximately two days before surgery	6 weeks / 6 months	6 weeks / 6 months	6 weeks / 6 months
			EQ-5D Index	0.56 ± 0.13	0.74 ± 0.16 / 0.79 ± 0.17	0.18 / 0.23	1.4 / 1.8
			Mobility	1.94 ± 0.27	1.56 ± 0.50 / 1.47 ± 0.50	0.38 / 0.47	1.4 / 1.7
			Self-care	2.02 + 0.49	1.60 ± 0.55 / 1.42 ± 0.51	0.42 / 0.60	0.9 / 1.2
			Usual activity	1.47 ± 0.57	1.24 ± 0.46 / 1.14 ± 0.35	0.23 / 0.33	0.4 / 0.6
			Pain/discomfort	2.20 ± 0.53	1.54 ± 0.51 / 1.45 ± 0.53	0.66 / 0.75	1.2 / 1.4
			Anxiety/depression	1.53 ± 0.57	1.20 ± 0.40 / 1.16 ± 0.37	0.33 / 0.37	0.6 / 0.6
Fielden et al, 2005, New Zealand[16]	Prospective observational; n = 122	OA, Women: 65%, Age: 66 (range, 35–85 years)	EQ-5D	Within month before surgery	1 month / 3 months / 6 months	1 month / 3 months / 6 months	Unable to calculate
			Mobility	1.97	1.85 / 1.30 / 1.30	0.00 / 1.30 / 1.30	
			Self-care	1.68	1.73 / 1.21 / 1.14	0.07 / 1.21 / 1.14	
			Usual activity	2.13	2.33 / 1.48 / 1.32	0.16 / 1.48 / 1.32	
			Pain/discomfort	2.33	1.81 / 1.48 / 1.38	0.10 / 1.48 / 1.38	
			Anxiety/depression	1.54	1.29 / 1.14 / 1.11	0.03 / 1.14 / 1.11	
Larsen et al, 2010, Denmark[56]	Prospective observational; n = 196	OA: NR, Women: 45%, Age: 70 ± 8.3 years	EQ-5D Index	1 week before surgery: 0.59 ± 0.23	3 months 0.84 ± 0.14 / 12 months 0.90 ± 0.14	3 months 0.25 / 12 months 0.31	3 months 1.1 / 12 months 1.3
Rasanen et al, 2007, Finland[55]	Prospective observational; n = 96	Primary arthritis 75%, Women: 63%, Age: 63 ± 12 years	15-D	NR: 0.81 ± 0.08	6 months 0.87 ± 0.09 / 12 months 0.86 ± 0.12	6 months 0.06 / 12 months 0.05	6 months 0.8 / 12 months 0.6

Study	Design	Demographics	n	Instrument	Preop Timepoint	Preop	Postop Timepoint	Postop	Change Timepoint	Change	Effect Size
Rolfson et al, 2009, Sweden[58]	Prospective observational	OA Women: 57% Age: 69 years (range, 27 to 96 years)	n = 6158	EQ-5D Index — Total	NR	0.39	1 year	0.77	1 year	0.38	Unable to calculate
				Men		0.44		0.80		0.36	
				Women		0.36		0.75		0.39	
Bachrach-Lindstrom et al, 2008, Sweden[13]	Prospective observational	OA Women: 48.9% Age: Men: 69 ± 10 years Women: 70 ± 10 years	n = 229	EQ-5D Index — Men	Within 1 week before surgery[a]	0.40 ± 0.03	1 year[a]	0.88 ± 0.02	1 year	0.48	Unable to calculate
				Women		0.37 ± 0.03		0.85 ± 0.02		0.48	
Ostendorf et al, 2004, Netherlands[25]	Prospective observational	OA: 83.3% Women: 62.3% Age: 67.6 ± 10.1 years	n = 114	EQ-5D Index	NR	0.35 ± 0.31	1 year	0.76 ± 0.27	1 year	0.41	1.3
				EQ-5D VAS		0.59 ± 0.22		0.75 ± 0.18		0.16	0.7
Lavernia et al, 2011, United States[59]	Prospective observational	OA: 45.9% Women: 53.1% Age: NR	n = 98	QWB Total Score	NR	0.52 ± 0.07	1 year	0.6 ± 0.1	1 year	0.08	1.1
Rolfson et al, 2011, Sweden[57]	Prospective observational	OA: 92.4% Women: 57.8% Age: 68.1 ± 10.4 years	n = 9727	EQ-5D Index	NR	0.41 ± 0.31	1 year	0.78 ± 024	1 year	0.37 ± 0.35	1.2
				EQ-5D VAS		54 ± 22		76 ± 20		22 ± 27	1.0
Quintana et al, 2005, Spain[26]	Prospective observational	OA Women: 50.7% Age: 69.4 ± 8.8 years	n = 469	SF-6D	While on waitlist	0.53 ± 0.13	6 months / 2 years	0.69 ± 0.16 / 0.71 ± 0.16	6 months / 2 years	0.16 / 0.18	6 months: 1.2 / 2 years: 1.4

Abbreviations: NR, not reported; OA, osteoarthritis; QWB, Quality of Well-Being; VAS, visual analog scale.

a Mean ± standard error.

with the SF-6D along with large effect sizes, 1.2 after six months, and 1.4 after 2 years.[26] Smaller effect sizes (ES = 0.6–0.8) were seen with the 15-D over 1 year in a smaller cohort.[55]

Total knee arthroplasty

Three studies used a utility measure to evaluate the effectiveness of TKA. A clinically important change in SF-6D score (0.11 units) was found 6 months after TKA (**Table 7**).[14] The 15-D detected a 0.02-point change at 6 months, which was not deemed a clinically important change[55]; however, gains at 12 months met the threshold of clinical importance (0.03).[55,60]

SUMMARY

A scoping review was completed to summarize the change in health status after THA and TKA. Although a recent study has performed a systematic review of functional recovery after THA,[61] we reviewed a broad topic of HRQL changes after total joint arthroplasty. This scoping review was not restricted by study design; however, the majority of studies were prospective single group, observational studies so that change over time could be reported. A variety of HRQL measures were used, including disease-specific, generic, and utility measures. We reported on 33 studies that met our inclusion criteria.

Most studies' primary outcomes were disease-specific measures. Not surprisingly, MCIDs were reported with recovery both short term and long term. These clinically relevant changes were accompanied with large effect sizes for pain and function using disease-specific measures such as the WOMAC. In general, smaller changes were reported with joint stiffness; however, this may also be related to inherent measurement properties of the WOMAC in that it uses two questions to evaluate stiffness. Overall, large effect sizes, in excess of 1.0, were seen not only short term but also long term, that is, more than a year after surgery. The changes may also be reflected in the low rate of complications reported with total joint arthroplasty.[62] The generic health measures showed a smaller magnitude of change, which is to be expected given the construct of these measures evaluate overall health and includes the effect of other health conditions. That being said, the largest changes were seen in those domains that were primary to total joint arthroplasty, pain and physical function.

A challenge of evaluating change of health status after total joint arthroplasty is that each measure has individual strengths and limitations. This review introduced the measures and the MCIDs when available to evaluate clinical change. The derived MCIDs should be considered carefully because these values are dependent on a number of features such as the study setting, methodology used to derive the values, baseline scores, and severity of the disease.[63] Change over time was also presented by the effect sizes. The effect size provided another perspective to measuring recovery after total joint arthroplasty in which comparison across measures can be made. Regardless of the type of outcome measure, large effect sizes are seen with total joint arthroplasty both over short-term and long-term outcomes.

Because a number of HRQL measures are used to evaluate the outcomes after total joint arthroplasties, comparisons can be challenging. This review summarized published findings to help place the magnitude of change seen with total joint arthroplasty in perspective. Changes seen with HRQL are one aspect of evaluating outcomes from a patient perspective; however, recovery is a complex concept[64] that needs many clinical and research-oriented measures to evaluate the full spectrum of recovery.

Table 7
Generic utility measures in total knee arthroplasty

Author, Year of Publication, Country	Study Design and Sample Size	Study Population	Measure/Domain	Baseline Mean (±SD) Score	Follow-up Mean (±SD) Score		Change		Effect Size	
					6 months	12 months	6 months	12 months	6 months	12 months
Escobar et al, 2007, Spain[14]	Prospective observational, n = 423	OA, Women: 75%, Age: 71.6 ± 6.7 years	SF-6D	NR, 0.55 ± 0.13	NR		0.11 ± 0.15		Unable to calculate	
Rasanen et al, 2007, Finland[55]	Prospective observational, n = 103	Primary arthritis: 90%, Women: 75%, Age: 69 ± 11 years	15-D	NR, 0.81 ± 0.09	0.83 ± 0.11	0.84 ± 0.11	0.02	0.03	0.2	0.3
Kauppila et al, 2011, Finland[60]	Prospective, single group, n = 88	OA, Women: 75%, Age: 70.7 ± 5.5 years	15-D	NR	NR		0.03 (95% CI: 0.02–0.05)		Unable to calculate	

Abbreviations: NR, not reported; OA, osteoarthritis.

ACKNOWLEDGMENTS

The authors thank Dale Storie, MLIS and Vania Gamache, MScPT for their assistance with this project, and also express their gratitude to Dr David Feeny for his constructive comments.

REFERENCES

1. Osoba D, King M. Meaningful differences. In: Fayers P, Hays R, editors. Assessing quality of life in clinical trials. 2nd edition. Oxford: Oxford University Press; 2005. p. 243–57.
2. Gossec L, Paternotte S, Maillefert JF, et al. The role of pain and functional impairment in the decision to recommend total joint replacement in hip and knee osteoarthritis: an international cross-sectional study of 1909 patients. Report of the OARSI-OMERACT Task Force on total joint replacement. Osteoarthritis Cartilage 2011;19(2):147–54.
3. Ritter MA, Albohm MJ. Overview: maintaining outcomes for total hip arthroplasty. The past, present, and future. Clin Orthop Relat Res 1997;(344):81–7.
4. Fitzpatrick R, Fletcher A, Gore S, et al. Quality of life measures in health care. I: Applications and issues in assessment. BMJ 1992;305(6861):1074–7.
5. Wilson IB, Kaplan S. Clinical practice and patients' health status: how are the two related? Med Care 1995;33(4 Suppl):AS209–14.
6. Riddle DL, Stratford PW, Bowman DH. Findings of extensive variation in the types of outcome measures used in hip and knee replacement clinical trials: a systematic review. Arthritis Rheum 2008;59(6):876–83.
7. Arksey H, O'Malley L. Scoping studies: towards a methodological framework. Int J Soc Res Method 2005;8(1):19–32.
8. Jaeschke R, Singer J, Guyatt GH. Measurement of health status: ascertaining the minimal clinically important difference. Control Clin Trials 1989;10(4):407–15.
9. Cohen J. A power primer. Psychol Bull 1992;112(1):155–9.
10. Bombardier C, Melfi CA, Paul J, et al. Comparison of a generic and a disease-specific measure of pain and physical function after knee replacement surgery. Med Care 1995;33(4 Suppl):AS131–44.
11. Dawson J, Fitzpatrick R, Murray D, et al. Comparison of measures to assess outcomes in total hip replacement surgery. Qual Health Care 1996;5(2):81–8.
12. Guyatt GH, Feeny DH, Patrick DL. Measuring health-related quality of life. Ann Intern Med 1993;118(8):622–9.
13. Bachrach-Lindstrom M, Karlsson S, Pettersson LG, et al. Patients on the waiting list for total hip replacement: a 1-year follow-up study. Scand J Caring Sci 2008;22(4):536–42.
14. Escobar A, Quintana JM, Bilbao A, et al. Responsiveness and clinically important differences for the WOMAC and SF-36 after total knee replacement. Osteoarthritis Cartilage 2007;15(3):273–80.
15. Escobar A, Quintana JM, Bilbao A, et al. Effect of patient characteristics on reported outcomes after total knee replacement. Rheumatology 2007;46(1):112–9.
16. Fielden JM, Cumming JM, Horne JG, et al. Waiting for hip arthroplasty: economic costs and health outcomes. J Arthroplasty 2005;20(8):990–7.
17. Fujita K, Makimoto K, Higo T, et al. Changes in the WOMAC, EuroQol and Japanese lifestyle measurements among patients undergoing total hip arthroplasty. Osteoarthritis Cartilage 2009;17(7):848–55.
18. Jones CA, Voaklander DC, Suarez-Alma ME. Determinants of function after total knee arthroplasty. Phys Ther 2003;83(8):696–706.

19. Kirschner S, Walther M, Bohm D, et al. German short musculoskeletal function assessment questionnaire (SMFA-D): comparison with the SF-36 and WOMAC in a prospective evaluation in patients with primary osteoarthritis undergoing total knee arthroplasty. Rheumatol Int 2003;23(1):15–20.

20. McQueen DA, Long MJ, Algotar AM, et al. The effect of obesity on quality-of-life improvement after total knee arthroplasty. Am J Orthop 2007;36(8):E117–20, E127.

21. Nilsdotter AK, Isaksson F. Patient relevant outcome 7 years after total hip replacement for OA: a prospective study. BMC Musculoskeletal Disord 2010;11:47.

22. Nunez M, Lozano L, Nunez E, et al. Total knee replacement and health-related quality of life: factors influencing long-term outcomes. Arthritis Rheumatism 2009;61(8): 1062–9.

23. Nunez M, Nunez E, Segur JM, et al. Health-related quality of life and costs in patients with osteoarthritis on waiting list for total knee replacement. Osteoarthritis Cartilage 2007;15(3):258–65.

24. Nunez M, Lozano L, Nunez E, et al. Good quality of life in severely obese total knee replacement patients: A case-control study. Obesity Surg 2011;21(8):1203–8.

25. Ostendorf M, van Stel HF, Buskens E, et al. Patient-reported outcome in total hip replacement: a comparison of five instruments of health status. J Bone Joint Surg [Br] 2004;86(6):801–8.

26. Quintana JM, Escobar A, Bilbao A, et al. Responsiveness and clinically important differences for the WOMAC and SF-36 after hip joint replacement. Osteoarthritis Cartilage 2005;13(12):1076–83.

27. SooHoo NF, Vyas RM, Samimi DB, et al. Comparison of the responsiveness of the SF-36 and WOMAC in patients undergoing total hip arthroplasty. J Arthroplasty 2007;22(8):1168–73.

28. Terwee CB, Van Der Slikke RMA, Van Lummel RC, et al. Self-reported physical functioning was more influenced by pain than performance-based physical functioning in knee-osteoarthritis patients. J Clin Epidemiol 2006;59(7):724–31.

29. Clement ND, Macdonald D, Howie CR, et al. The outcome of primary total hip and knee arthroplasty in patients aged 80 years or more. J Bone Joint Surg [Br] 2011; 93(9):1265–70.

30. Ko Y, Narayanasamy S, Wee H-L, et al. Health-related quality of life after total knee replacement or unicompartmental knee arthroplasty in an urban Asian population. Value Health 2011;14(2):322–8.

31. Xie F, Lo NN, Pullenayegum EM, et al. Evaluation of health outcomes in osteoarthritis patients after total knee replacement: a two-year follow-up. Health Qual Life Outcomes 2010;8:87.

32. Uesugi Y, Makimoto K, Fujita K. Validity and responsiveness of the Oxford Hip Score in a prospective study with Japanese total hip arthroplasty patients. J Orthop Sci 2009;14(1):35–9.

33. Murray DW, Fitzpatrick R, Rogers K, et al. The use of the Oxford Hip and Knee scores. J Bone Joint Surg [Br] 2007;89(8):1010–4.

34. March LM, Barcenilla AL, Cross MJ, et al. Costs and outcomes of total hip and knee joint replacement for rheumatoid arthritis. Clin Rheumatol 2008;27(10):1235–42.

35. Bellamy N. WOMAC Osteoarthritis Index User Guide IX. 2009.

36. Bruce B, Fries JF. The Stanford Health Assessment Questionnaire: dimensions and practical applications. Health Qual Life Outcomes 2003;1:20.

37. Ware JE Jr. SF-36 health survey update. Spine (Phila 1976) 2000;25(24):3130–9.

38. Ware J Jr, Kosinski M, Keller SD. A 12-item short-form health survey: construction of scales and preliminary tests of reliability and validity. Med Care 1996;34(3):220–33.

39. Busija L, Osborne RH, Nilsdotter A, et al. Magnitude and meaningfulness of change in SF-36 scores in four types of orthopedic surgery. Health Qual Life Outcomes 2008;6:55.

40. Zeni J, Axe M, Snyder-Mackler L. The Delaware Osteoarthritis Profile: a comprehensive evaluation of disability and recovery. Osteoarthritis Cartilage Conference: 2010 Osteoarthritis Research Society International, OARSI World Congress Brussels Belgium, September 23–26, 2010; 18S132–3.

41. Hunt SM, McEwen J. The development of a subjective health indicator. Sociol Health Illn 1980;2(3):231–46.

42. Koivunen K, Sintonen H, Lukkarinen H. Properties of the 15D and the Nottingham Health Profile questionnaires in patients with lower limb atherosclerotic disease. Int J Technol Assess Health Care 2007;23(3):385–91.

43. Bergner M, Bobbitt RA, Carter WB, et al. The Sickness Impact Profile: development and final revision of a health status measure. Med Care 1981;19(8):787–805.

44. MacKenzie CR, Charlson ME, DiGioia D, et al. Can the sickness impact profile measure change? An example of scale assessment. J Chronic Dis 1986;39(6):429–38.

45. Shi HY, Khan M, Culbertson R, et al. Health-related quality of life after total hip replacement: a Taiwan study. Int Orthop 2009;33(5):1217–22.

46. Badura-Brzoza K, Zajac P, Brzoza Z, et al. Psychological and psychiatric factors related to health-related quality of life after total hip replacement—preliminary report. Eur Psychiatry 2009;24(2):119–24.

47. Montin L, Suominen T, Haaranen E, et al. The changes in health-related quality of life and related factors during the process of total hip arthroplasty. Int J Nurs Pract 2011;17(1):19–26.

48. Dowsey MM, Liew D, Stoney JD, et al. The impact of obesity on weight change and outcomes at 12 months in patients undergoing total hip arthroplasty. Med J Aust 2010;193(1):17–21.

49. Tsonga T, Kapetanakis S, Papadopoulos C, et al. Evaluation of improvement in quality of life and physical activity after total knee arthroplasty in Greek elderly women. Orthop J 2011;5:343–7.

50. Peterlein CD, Schofer MD, Fuchs-Winkelmann S, et al. Clinical outcome and quality of life after computer-assisted total knee arthroplasty: results from a prospective, single-surgeon study and review of the literature. Musculoskeletal Surg 2009;93(3):115–22.

51. O'Brien BJ, Spath M, Blackhouse G, et al. A view from the bridge: agreement between the SF-6D utility algorithm and the Health Utilities Index. Health Econ 2003;12(11):975–81.

52. Feeny D. A utility approach to the assessment of health-related quality of life. Med Care 2000;38(9 Suppl):II1514.

53. Kopec JA, Willison KD. A comparative review of four preference-weighted measures of health-related quality of life. J Clin Epidemiol 2003;56(4):317–25.

54. Sintonen H. The 15D instrument of health-related quality of life: properties and applications. Ann Med 2001;33(5):328–36.

55. Rasanen P, Paavolainen P, Sintonen H, et al. Effectiveness of hip or knee replacement surgery in terms of quality-adjusted life years and costs. Acta Orthop 2007;78(1):108–15.

56. Larsen K, Hansen TB, Soballe K, et al. Patient-reported outcome after fast-track hip arthroplasty: a prospective cohort study. Health Qual Life Outcomes 2010;8:144.

57. Rolfson O, Karrholm J, Dahlberg LE, et al. Patient-reported outcomes in the Swedish Hip Arthroplasty Register: results of a nationwide prospective observational study. J Bone Joint Surg [Br] 2011;93(7):867–75.

58. Rolfson O, Dahlberg LE, Nilsson JA, et al. Variables determining outcome in total hip replacement surgery. J Bone Joint Surg [Br] 2009;91(2):157–61.

59. Lavernia CJ, Alcerro JC. Quality of life and cost-effectiveness 1 year after total hip arthroplasty. J Arthroplasty 2011;26(5):705–9.
60. Kauppila AM, Kyllonen E, Ohtonen P, et al. Outcomes of primary total knee arthroplasty: the impact of patient-relevant factors on self-reported function and quality of life. Disabil Rehabil 2011;33(17–18):1659–67.
61. Vissers MM, Bussmann JB, Verhaar JA, et al. Recovery of physical functioning after total hip arthroplasty: systematic review and meta-analysis of the literature. Phys Ther 2011;91(5):615–29.
62. Singh JA, Kwoh CK, Boudreau RM, et al. Hospital volume and surgical outcomes after elective hip/knee arthroplasty: a risk-adjusted analysis of a large regional database. Arthritis Rheum 2011;63(8):2531–9.
63. Wells G, Beaton D, Shea B, et al. Minimal clinically important differences: review of methods. J Rheumatol 2001;28(2):406–12.
64. Beaton DE, Tarasuk V, Katz JN, et al. "Are you better?" A qualitative study of the meaning of recovery. Arthritis Rheum 2001;45(3):270–9.

Revision Total Hip and Knee Replacement

Andrew J. Barnett, MRCS (Ed), FRCS (Trauma & Orth)*,
Andrew D. Toms, MSc, FRCS (Trauma & Orth), FRCS (Ed)

KEYWORDS

- Revision • Total hip replacement • Total knee replacement • Indications
- Outcome • Complications

KEY POINTS

- The number of primary and revision total joint arthroplasty procedures is increasing exponentially with time. It is anticipated that there will be a huge expected demand for revision knee surgery over the next 2 decades. Knee revisions alone are projected to increase by 601% between 2005 and 2030 in the United States.
- Awareness is needed by both general practitioner and physician for the signs of failure of these implants and when to refer on to the surgeon. Infection remains the primary cause to exclude first. Unless the surgeon accurately identifies the mode of failure, successful treatment becomes very unlikely; an increasing physical burden on the patient and financial burden on hospital trusts ensues.
- In comparison with primary joint arthroplasty, complication rates after revision surgery are significantly increased and outcome less assured.

INTRODUCTION

Total hip replacement (THR) and total knee replacement (TKR) are undoubtedly two of the most successful operations performed today. Owing to an increasingly elderly population, better medical care, improved implant design, and consumer pressure, numbers of primary and revision hip and knee replacements continue to increase. In 2010, 68,907 primary THR and 81,979 primary TKRs were performed in the United Kingdom.[1] In the same year, 7,852 revision THRs and 5,082 revision TKRs were performed. Kurtz and colleagues[2] have shown that the demand for revision total hip and total knee revisions is projected to grow by 137% and 601%, respectively, between 2005 and 2030 in the United States. Revision procedures represent a significant burden for patients, their treating physician, and surgeon and are also a financial burden for hospital trusts. This population has greater expectations and

Exeter Knee Reconstruction Unit, Royal Devon and Exeter Hospital, Barrack Road, Exeter, EX2 5DW, UK
* Corresponding author.
E-mail address: andybarnett60@hotmail.com

Clin Geriatr Med 28 (2012) 431–446
http://dx.doi.org/10.1016/j.cger.2012.05.008
0749-0690/12/$ – see front matter © 2012 Elsevier Inc. All rights reserved.

Table 1	
Mode of failure	
THR	**TKR**
Infection	Infection
Aseptic loosening	Aseptic loosening
Dislocation	Tibio-femoral instability
Periprosthetic fracture	Periprosthetic fracture
Implant breakage (rare)	Extensor mechanism rupture
	Patellar complications/component malrotation
	Implant breakage (rare)

multiple comorbidities presenting a greater risk for a major surgical procedure. This article aims to clarify the modes of failure of hip and knee replacements, when to refer to a surgeon, surgical considerations for revision, outcome, and complications.

MODES OF FAILURE

The overall survivorship of THR and TKR is approximately 90% at 15 years, depending on the type of implant used. When joint replacements fail, they may require a revision procedure to exchange the implants. One common myth is that patients may only have 1 revision procedure during their lifetime; however, this simply is not the case. There is no limit to the number of revision procedures a patient may have, assuming there is an appropriate indication, and the patient is medically fit. The common modes of failure of THR and TKR are discussed below (**Table 1**).

Infection

Deep infection after total joint arthroplasty is a devastating complication. The incidence after TKR or THR is approximately 1%, so it is relatively rare; however, it results in significant suffering for patients. There are a number of risk factors for infection, including diabetes, obesity, rheumatoid arthritis, sickle cell disease, human immunodeficiency virus infection, malignancy, and immunosuppression.

Infection can be classified as acute or chronic. Acute infections, the majority of which represent infection acquired at the time of operation, occur within the first month after surgery, whereas chronic infection presents months or years later. Chronic infections are caused by hematogenous spread of organisms, months or years after the original operation.

The diagnosis of infection requires a high index of clinical suspicion. There is no single reliable test, but a combined approach using the quadruple assessment of clinical evaluation, serologic investigation, diagnostic imaging, and microbiologic analysis should enable the diagnosis of infection to be made with a high degree of confidence.[3]

Staphylococcus aureus, Staphylococcus epidermidis, and coliforms are the most common organisms responsible. Some bacteria produce a glycocalyx, which functions as a biofilm. This biofilm helps bacteria adhere to the implant and inhibits macrophages and protects them from antibiotics. Most commonly, this requires 2 operations (2-stage revision procedure) to eradicate the infection. The first operation involves removing the joint replacement and excising all infected tissue. A temporary joint replacement (made of antibiotic-laden cement) is implanted to allow the patient

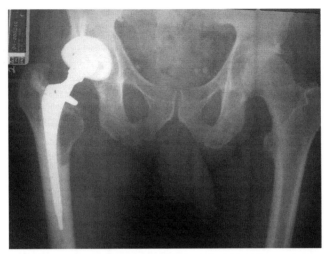

Fig. 1. AP radiograph of the pelvis shows wear particle-induced osteolysis around a right total hip replacement.

to mobilize and return home on oral antibiotics. The second operation is then planned to permanently reconstruct the joint, which is performed when the soft tissues have settled and the infection has cleared. Generally, the second operation is undertaken when the C-reactive protein has normalized.

Aseptic Loosening

Aseptic loosening is the most common cause of failure of THR and the second most common cause of failure in TKR. When a cobalt chrome femoral head articulates with a polyethylene cup, tiny wear particles (diameter 0.3–10 μm) are produced, which activate macrophages. In turn, these macrophages release cytokines, prostaglandins, and tumor necrosis factor, which not only cause osteolysis but also stimulate osteoclastic bone resorption (**Fig. 1**). The end result is cement-bone interface loosening. In addition to polyethylene wear particles, metallic, cement, and ceramic particles may also incite a host response leading to bony destruction (osteolysis).

Dislocation/Instability

The dislocation rate after primary THR is reported to be 1% to 3% (**Fig. 2**). The etiology of dislocation may be classified as patient related, surgeon related, and implant related. Rates of dislocation are highest within the first 3 months after surgery. When dislocation becomes recurrent, revision surgery often becomes necessary. The initial treatment is with closed reduction then treatment in a brace. After a second or third dislocation, patients are normally offered revision surgery, and constrained acetabular components can be used, which reduce the risk of further dislocation.

Dislocation after TKR is fortunately a rare occurrence. Instability, however, is increasingly recognized as a mode of failure and can be very disabling. The main options for treatment of instability are isolated polyethylene spacer exchange or full component revision using a more constrained knee replacement or hinged knee. Constrained implants help stabilize the knee in 2 planes. They provide antero-posterior (AP) as well as varus/valgus stability and are used mainly in cases of

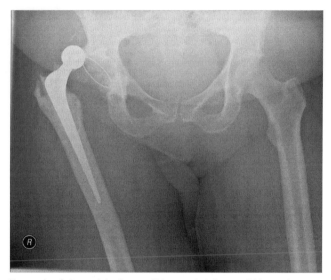

Fig. 2. AP radiograph of the pelvis shows dislocated right total hip replacement.

collateral ligament insufficiency. Hinged knee replacements are generally used in cases of instability associated with significant bone loss in addition to collateral ligament insufficiency. **Fig. 3** illustrates the differences between primary TKR and hinged knee replacement components. Periprosthetic fracture data from the Swedish Hip Registry has shown that after THR, periprosthetic femoral fractures were the third most common cause for reoperation (9.5%) after aseptic loosening (60.1%) and recurrent

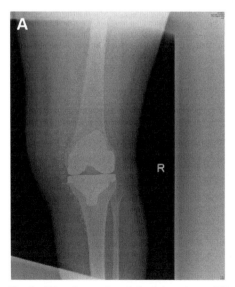
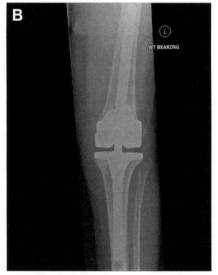

Fig. 3. AP radiographs of the knee show differences between primary TKR (A) and hinged TKR (B).

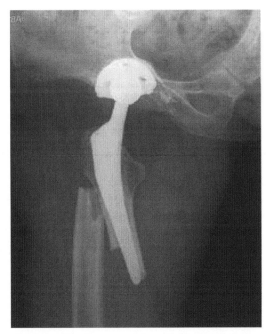

Fig. 4. AP radiograph of the hip shows a periprosthetic fracture around an uncemented femoral stem.

dislocation (13.1%).[4] These fractures may occur intraoperatively or postoperatively. Intraoperative fractures are more likely to occur when using uncemented implants (**Fig. 4**). Meek and coworkers[5] report the overall rate of fracture was 0.9% after primary THR, 4.2% after revision THR, 0.6% after primary TKR, and 1.7% after revision TKR. The femur is much more commonly fractured in both THR and TKR. Postoperative fractures may occur after major trauma or more commonly as a result of minor trauma in combination with osteoporosis or loose implant.

RISK FACTORS FOR REVISION TOTAL HIP AND KNEE REPLACEMENT

The risk factors for revision joint replacement may be classified into modifiable and nonmodifiable. These are summarized in **Table 2** below.

WHEN TO REFER TO AN ORTHOPEDIC SURGEON

When hip and knee replacements start to fail, the most common symptom is pain. In the case of deep infection, the pain is constant and deep seated and worsens with activity; very often pain will have been present from the start. If the wound looks clearly infected or there has been wound breakdown, the diagnosis is a straightforward one, although this is rarely the case. Raised inflammatory markers in the absence of any other source of infection also raise suspicion of infection. If the C-reactive protein (CRP) and erythrocyte sedimentation rate (ESR) levels are both elevated, the probability of infection has been noted to be 83%, whereas if they are both negative, infection can be reliably excluded.[3,6] If in any doubt, all patients with possible infection should be referred on to an orthopedic surgeon. It is important that antibiotics should not be commenced until they have been seen by the surgeon; there

Table 2	
Risk factors for revision joint replacement	
Modifiable	**Nonmodifiable**
Inadequate aseptic precautions during surgery	Youthfulness
Technical incompetence	Male sex
Prolonged operating time	Primary joint replacement for trauma, eg, after pelvic or femoral fracture
Component malposition	Primary joint replacement for osteoarthritis secondary to childhood disorders, eg, Perthe's disease, developmental dysplasia of the hip
Poor cementing technique	Rheumatoid arthritis
Faulty implant	
Poor implant design	
Obesity	
Increased physical activity	

is a high incidence of false-negative joint aspiration in the presence of concurrent antibiotic use.[7]

A history of start-up pain (eg, getting out of a chair) is a classic presentation of a loose component secondary to a number of modes of failure including aseptic and septic loosening. Buttock pain suggests a loose cup, whereas thigh pain indicates femoral component loosening. Loosening of any cause is commonly associated with an initial sharp exacerbation of pain when a patient first stands, which steadily reduces with mobilization. Radiographs may clearly reveal the diagnosis of osteolysis and component loosening (see **Fig. 1**) or, as in the case of TKR, changes may be difficult to identify. With or without radiographic findings, this history requires referral.

Progressive limb shortening or a limp with an associated reduction in exercise tolerance or reliance on walking aids should prompt referral as should any history of instability whether resolved or ongoing.

Symptoms and signs of a failing joint replacement include the following:

- New-onset increasing pain following pain-free period after joint replacement
- Worsening pain and reduced exercise tolerance
- Loss of mobility and increased reliance on walking aids
- Increasing stiffness
- Limb shortening and increased limp
- Joint instability.

PREOPERATIVE EVALUATION

The results from primary TKR and THR are generally excellent with reproducible success rates in more than 90% of patients at 10-year follow-up. As discussed earlier, there are numerous modes of failure leading to the need for revision total joint arthroplasty (TJR). Revision TJR is far more challenging for the surgeon to perform with higher risks and poorer outcome. Despite the increased risks associated with revision surgery, advanced age should not preclude patients from surgery, assuming they are medically fit. To optimize success, thorough preoperative evaluation and planning is essential. Most importantly, the surgeon must determine why and how the implant failed.

| **Box 1** |
| **Key questions to ask patient with a troublesome joint replacement** |

Was it good initially and then started causing problems?

Was it bad right from the start?

Were there any problems with the wound healing after surgery?

Any history of chest/urinary/dental sepsis?

Does the joint feel stable/any episodes of instability?

Any history of recurrent knee swelling?

Do you get pain getting out of a chair that settles as you mobilize further?

Evaluation of the patient with a problematic joint replacement requires a thorough history and clinical examination, imaging, and laboratory tests.

History

It is important to accurately define the nature of the patient's pain. This includes the location, severity, duration, and any exacerbating or relieving factors. Pain that develops years after TJR is suggestive of component wear or loosening, ligamentous instability, or a hematogenous infection. In contrast, when the TJR was never pain free, diagnoses such as infection, instability, and referred pain (radiation of pain from another joint) should be considered. The surgeon must exclude conditions in which TJR may be contraindicated (eg, Charcot arthropathy, neuromuscular disease, psychiatric illness, active sepsis, and serious systemic disease).

Patients with hip subluxation often describe "clicking," "popping," or a feeling of the hip moving in and out of joint. For those patients who have experienced dislocation, the number of episodes and the position of the limb at the time of dislocation are important in decision making. **Box 1** summarizes the key questions to ask in the history.

Physical Examination

Clinical examination is equally important in the complete clinical workup. The skin overlying the joint is inspected for old scars and sinuses. Limb length and alignment, range of joint motion, ligamentous stability, and patellar tracking should all be assessed. It is essential to examine the joint above and the joint below to exclude referred pain. Spinal stenosis or high lumbar disc pathology may present with hip and anterior knee pain. A positive femoral stretch test will help identify a high lumbar radiculopathy as a source of knee pain. Knee pain is also commonly caused by ipsilateral hip arthritis or vascular disease. These can be ruled out with clinical examination and subsequent imaging.

A neurologic examination is necessary to ensure the patient has adequate motor control of the lower limb and also to exclude any neurologic disease. Significant peripheral vascular disease is a relative contraindication to revision surgery, and peripheral pulses must be checked. If in doubt, vascular studies or a preoperative vascular consultation should be organized. **Table 3** shows the differential diagnoses of a painful THR or THK.

Table 3 Differential diagnosis of a painful THR/TKA	
THR	**TKR**
Lumbar spine arthritis	Hip osteoarthritis
Spinal stenosis	Lumbar spine arthritis
Sciatica	Spinal stenosis
Peripheral vascular disease	High lumbar radiculopathy
Malignancy	Peripheral vascular disease
Stress fractures	Malignancy
	Stress fractures

Imaging

Routine imaging of the affected hip should include an AP pelvis and a lateral radiograph. When imaging the knee, AP, lateral, and skyline views (imaging the patellofemoral articulation) should be obtained.

All radiographs should be examined carefully to assess component fixation and position, evidence of significant deformity, loosening, bone loss, and infection (periosteal reaction). Definite loosening of cemented implants exists if significant or progressive component migration is seen (eg, femoral stem subsidence or cement mantle fracture; a continuous radiolucent line at the bone-cement interface indicates probable loosening; and evidence of a radiolucent of 50% to 99% at the bone-cement interface indicates possible loosening).[8,9]

Laboratory Tests

To rule out infection, a full blood count, CRP and ESR blood tests are performed. Assessment of the white blood cell count is of limited benefit, as it is often normal.[3] It is important to bear in mind that in the uncomplicated arthroplasty, CRP levels return to normal within the first 3 weeks after operation, whereas the ESR may take up to 1 year to normalize.[10] Joint aspiration also aids diagnosis. Barrack and colleagues[11] looked at the value of knee aspiration in determining infection in 69 cases of revision TKR. They found a sensitivity of 65.4% and a specificity of 96.1%. Mason and coworkers[12] examined the preoperative knee aspirates of 86 patients who underwent revision TKR. They analyzed white cell count and percentage of polymorphonucleocytes. Aspirates containing greater than 2,500 white blood cells per high-power field in conjunction with greater than 60% polymorphonucleocytes indicated a high likelihood of infection. The authors demonstrated a sensitivity of 98% and a specificity of 95% for diagnosis of infection using these criteria.

SURGICAL TECHNIQUE

The goals of revision surgery are to remove the failed prosthesis, insert new components with the aim of providing long-term rigid, stable fixation, and, if possible, augment deficient bone stock. Where possible, these aims are achieved using the original surgical incision, although this often requires extension. With a failed TKA, in the rare situation of multiple longitudinal incisions being present, it is wise to use the most lateral incision to minimize vascular compromise to overlying skin.

In the case of a stiff TKA, exposure of the knee joint may require a "rectus snip" (**Fig. 5**) or a tibial tubercle osteotomy. The latter procedure requires either screw

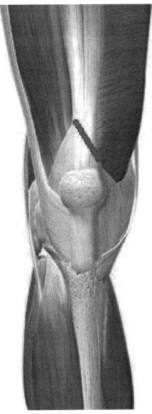

Fig. 5. Schematic diagram shows the rectus snip approach to enhance exposure during TKR.

or wire fixation afterward and introduces the possibility of nonunion.[13] With a rectus snip, in addition to the standard medial arthrotomy to access the knee joint (medial parapatellar approach), the quadriceps is divided at a 45° angle. This has been shown to have no adverse effect on functional outcome.[14]

Specific to the hip, an extended trochanteric osteotomy is sometimes required to aid stem and cement removal,[15] which again adds the risk of nonunion. When reimplanting, the stem of the revision implant needs to bypass the osteotomy site by a length of 2 cortical diameters, otherwise the risk of periprosthetic fracture is significantly increased. After adequate exposure, it is essential to remove any loose cement, debris, and granulation tissue before reimplantation. An assessment of bone loss will then determine the subsequent means of hip/knee reconstruction. Revision is generally performed in 2 stages for infection (separated by a minimum of 6 weeks) or 1 stage for most other indications.

Hip Reconstruction

Reconstruction consists of either a cemented or uncemented approach for both the acetabulum and femur.

Acetabular reconstruction

The goals of acetabular reconstruction are to achieve stable fixation of the prosthesis, restore the anatomic center of hip rotation, and to correct bone deficiency.[16] Using cemented revision components, it is often necessary to use bone graft to improve the quality of fixation at the cement–bone interface. Bony defects can be reconstructed using mesh, structural allograft, or trabecular metal wedges. Larger defects can be addressed with an uncemented cup, which relies on a press-fit for fixation, often supplemented with screws. The porous outer surface of the cup is coated with hydroxyapatite, which encourages long-term biological fixation by encouraging bony ongrowth or ingrowth, depending on design. In cases of very significant bone loss, trabecular metal cups, with an outer surface resembling the structure of cancellous bone can be used. With these cups, ingrowth occurs quickly, and long-term fixation may be stronger. Supplementary plate fixation or acetabular cages are used to treat pelvic discontinuity, where progressive bone loss leads to separation of the superior and inferior parts of the pelvis.[17]

Femoral reconstruction

When the cement–bone interface remains intact, and the femoral side is not the cause for revision, an in-cement revision can be performed. This involves cementing a smaller stem into the old cement mantle and has good medium-term results.[18] When the cement mantle is of poor quality, it requires removal. Without supplementary bone grafting of the femur, cemented revision has poor long-term results; the revised cement–bone interface has been shown to be 80% weaker than that in primary THR.[19] Instead, femoral impaction grafting is often used by surgeons to improve the quality of the bone–cement interface. This method utilizes morselized allograft bone impacted into the proximal femur and has excellent 10-year results.[20] If reconstruction of the proximal femur is not possible, an uncemented femoral stem relying on distal fixation may be used be used to bypass the defect. Uncemented implants are an increasingly popular choice because they are quicker to implant, they are more straightforward to perform than impaction grafting, and their modular nature provides more flexibility in positioning the femoral head. Their use does carry an increased risk of femoral fracture and perforation; however, in the absence of these complications, there is no significant difference between uncemented and cemented implants from a functional point of view.

Knee Reconstruction

The choice of implant depends on the indication for revision and the degree of bone and soft tissue destruction after implant removal. There are a range of different implants available depending on the degree of constraint required and size of the bony defect. At the top of the constraint ladder is the hinged knee replacement, which caters for severe distal femoral bone loss with loss of ligamentous attachment. As the degree of constraint increases, the shear stress at the component–bone interface also increases. To decrease this stress, femoral and tibial stems are used to increase the area of implant fixation and spread the load.

In both hip and knee reconstruction, when there is massive bone loss, femoral and/or tibial replacing "megaprostheses" may be used (**Fig. 6**); these function best in elderly, low-demand patients.

MANAGEMENT OF DEEP INFECTION IN TOTAL HIP AND KNEE ARTHROPLASTY

Despite significant advances in surgical technique and perioperative care, the incidence of deep infection in total joint arthroplasty is generally quoted as being 1%.

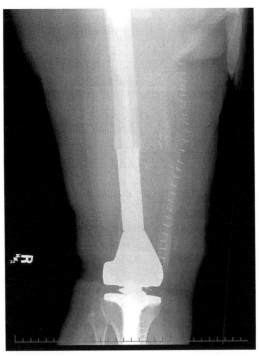

Fig. 6. AP radiograph of the femur shows distal femoral replacement in situ after revision TKR complicated by significant bone loss.

Having diagnosed a deep infection there are a number of therapeutic options available to the surgeon managing this devastating complication. The options are:

- Suppressive antibiotic therapy
- Surgical debridement with retention of the components
- Single-stage revision
- Two-stage revision
- Arthrodesis (fusion)
- Girdlestone procedure (hip only).

The treatment option depends on a number of factors, including patient fitness, complexity of the surgery, and the severity of the infection.[3] Suppressive antibiotic therapy is generally reserved for patients who either do not want further surgery or are deemed unfit. The components must be well fixed and the isolated organism (generally of low-virulence) sensitive to the antibiotic being used. Analysis of the literature reveals that this option is successful in only 21% of patients.[21]

For infections occurring within 1 month of the original procedure, surgical debridement with retention of well-fixed components has been shown to yield success rates of approximately 30%.[22] After this 1-month "window of opportunity" the chance of successfully eradicating infection falls significantly.

In patients presenting with chronic deep infection, the exchange surgery can be performed as either a single-stage or 2-stage revision. The gold standard treatment is a 2-stage revision with high recurrence rates as low as 5.6%.[23] This involves 2 major operations and a significant length of hospital stay, and the patient mobilizes with a

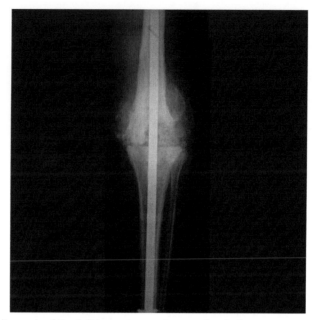

Fig. 7. AP radiograph of the left knee shows a knee arthrodesis.

temporary joint replacement often made from cement loaded with antibiotics. The second-stage procedure is generally performed a minimum of 6 weeks after the first stage when the CRP has normalized.

In cases in which there is an isolated infecting organism with known antibiotic sensitivities and a fit patient without comorbidities that affect their ability to fight infection, a single-stage revision can be performed. This has implications for both the patient and the treating hospital. Both hospital stay and costs are dramatically reduced, and this scenario may be beneficial to the patient both physically and psychologically.

If, after debridement, the patient either declines further surgery or hip reconstruction is not possible, then resection arthroplasty is a viable option. Although the chances of eradicating infection are high, lower limb function is poor. In both failed hip and knee arthoplasties, an arthrodesis may be performed (**Fig. 7**). This is when the joint is fused in a position of function with the aim of providing a stiff but pain-free and stable limb upon which to mobilize.

Disarticulation is reserved for life-threatening sepsis or irreparable neurovascular damage around the hip and is used as a last resort.

COMPLICATIONS OF REVISION TOTAL HIP AND KNEE ARTHROPLASTY

Revision total joint arthroplasty is a major undertaking associated with increased operating time and significant blood loss. Owing to the complexity of these procedures, the complication rate is considerably higher than in that seen with primary total joint arthroplasty. **Table 4** lists these complications and their incidence.

OUTCOME AFTER REVISION TOTAL HIP AND KNEE REPLACEMENT

Outcome depends on the type of revision procedure performed and the indication for surgery. This makes it difficult to compare different studies and also to make

Table 4
Complications after revision total hip and knee replacement (incidence in parentheses)

	Revision THR	Revision TKR
Intraoperative	Nerve injury (1.4%)	Nerve injury (0.6%)
	Vascular injury (0.08%)	Vascular injury (0.17%)
	Fracture (7%)	Fracture (1%)
		Patella tendon avulsion
Postoperative	Infection (1%)	Infection (1%)
	Dislocation (8%)	Dislocation (rare)
	Fracture (4.2%)	Fracture (1.7%)
	DVT/PE (1.8%)	DVT/PE (1.4%)
	Heterotopic ossification (3%–7%)	

generalizations about outcome overall. Undoubtedly, however, outcome after revision joint replacement is not as favorable as primary joint replacement.

RESULTS OF REVISION TOTAL HIP REPLACEMENT
Patient-Related Outcome

Revision total hip arthroplasty has a higher complication rate than primary arthroplasty; patients are older and surgery is more technically demanding. These factors combine to produce a poorer outcome.[24] One study from Robinson and coworkers[25] found no difference in pain scores between revision THR and primary THR, but function deteriorated significantly in the former group. Saleh and colleagues[26] performed a meta-analysis of functional outcome after revision hip arthroplasty. This revealed slightly higher morbidity and mortality rates than primary hip replacement and slightly lower functional outcome using global hip scores.

Biring and colleagues[27] looked at predictors of quality-of-life outcomes after revision THR. They found that all patients' quality-of-life scores improved after surgery and that a higher preoperative function score, age between 60 and 70 years, male sex, and the indication for revision being aseptic loosening were all predictive of improved outcome after surgery.

Surgical-Related Outcome

Acetabular component revision
Results for acetabular component revision alone vary from a 0% reoperation rate using cementless components at 44 months[28] to 22% at 14- to 20-year follow-up using cemented techniques.[29]

Femoral component revision
Katz and coworkers[29] found higher success rates with their cemented femoral revisions. Their rerevision rate at 14- to 20-year follow-up was only 5%. In certain situations, a cement-in-cement technique can be used to revise the femoral component, when there is an intact cement mantle and bone–cement interface. Excellent results have been shown with no stem loosening after 5 years.[30]

Outcome of Revision Total Hip Replacement for Infection

Two-stage revision has long been regarded the gold standard for treating infection. Haddad and colleagues[31] reported a reinfection rate of 8% at 5-year follow-up using this technique.

RESULTS OF REVISION TOTAL KNEE REPLACEMENT

Before the early 1990s, there was a lack of available literature, and any published studies tended to comprise small numbers and short follow-up with high complication rates. More recently, long-term results of modern revision techniques have become available but not in the numbers seen with revision THR.

Patient-Related Outcome

Friedman and colleagues[32] reported that pain levels, range of motion, instability, and function all improved after aseptic revision TKR; however, these improvements were significantly less than in those who underwent primary TKR. Hanssen and coworkers,[33] when comparing revision and primary TKR, found 92% good or excellent results in the primary TKR group but only 81% after revision TKR.

Wang and colleagues[34] reported the clinical outcome and patient satisfaction in aseptic and septic revision TKRs. In the aseptic group, 79% reported their result as excellent compared with only 33% in the septic group. In addition, the aseptic revisions had better range of motion and knee scores, whereas their functional and knee scores were similar.

Surgical-Related Outcome

Murray and colleagues[35] published one of the earliest large series of cemented revision TKRs. At a mean follow-up of 58 months, there was 1 femoral loosening and no loose tibial components in 40 revision TKRs. This study set the benchmark for which all other similar studies are compared. Whaley and colleagues[36] reviewed 38 cemented revision TKRs; the 11-year survivorship for aseptic loosening was 96%.

Gofton and coworkers[37] reported 89 revisions using uncemented components with a mean follow-up of 5.9 years. There were 7 cases of rerevision for aseptic loosening and a 94% survivorship at 8.6 years.

Fehring and coworkers[38] published the only study comparing cemented and uncemented fixation in revision TKR. In the cemented group, 93% of components were stable compared with only 71% in the uncemented group. The authors expressed concerns about the use of cementless components in revision TKR.

Outcome of Revision Total Knee Replacement for Infection

As with revision THR, the deep infection rate after revision TKR is significantly increased. Hanssen and colleagues[39] published a study of 89 infected TKRs that were treated with a number of different protocols over a 10-year period. At mean follow-up of 52 months, the rate of recurrent infection was 11%, whereas the overall complication was 34%.

SUMMARY

The number of primary and revision total joint arthroplasty procedures is increasing exponentially with time. It is anticipated that there will be a huge expected demand for revision knee surgery over the next 2 decades. Knee revisions alone are projected to increase by 601% between 2005 and 2030 in the United States.[2] Awareness is needed by both general practitioner and physician for the signs of failure of these implants and when to refer to the surgeon. Infection remains the primary cause to exclude first. Unless the surgeon accurately identifies the mode of failure, successful treatment becomes very unlikely; an increasing physical burden on the patient and financial burden on hospital trusts ensues. In comparison with primary joint arthroplasty, complication rates after revision surgery are significantly increased, and outcome is less assured.

REFERENCES

1. UK National Joint Registry data, 2010.
2. Kurtz S, Ong K, Lau E, et al. Projections of primary revision hip and knee arthroplasty in the United States from 2005 to 2030. J Bone Joint Surg Am 2007;89:780–5.
3. Toms AD, Davidson D, Masri BA, et al. The management of periprosthetic infection in total joint arthroplasty. J Bone Surg Br 2006;88–B:149–55.
4. Lindahl H, Malchau H, Herberts P, et al. Periprosthetic femoral fractures classification and demographics of 1049 periprosthetic fractures from the Swedish National Hip Arthroplasty Register. J Arthroplasty 2005;20(7):857–65.
5. Meek MD, Norwood T, Smith R, et al. The risk of peri-prosthetic fracture after primary and revision total hip and knee replacement. J Bone Joint Surg Br 2011;93–B:96–101.
6. Spangehl MJ, Masri BA, O'Connell JX, et al. Prospective analysis of preoperative and intraoperative investigations for the diagnosis of infection at the sites of two hundred and tow revision total hip arthroplasties. J Bone Joint Surg Am 1999;81(A):672–83.
7. Barrack RL. The value of preoperative knee aspiration: don't ask, don't tell. Orthopedics 1997;20:862–4.
8. Harris WH, McCarthy JC Jr, O'Neill DA. Femoral component loosening using contemporary techniques of femoral cement fixation. J Bone J Surg Am 1982;64:1063–7.
9. Johnston RC, Fitzgerald RH Jr, Harris WH, et al. Clinical and radiographic evaluation of total hip replacement. A Standard system of terminology for reporting results. J Bone Joint Surg Am 1990;72:161–8.
10. Shin LY, Wu JJ, Yang DJ. Eryrthocyte sedimentation rate and C-reactive protein values in patients with total hip arthroplasty. Clin Orthop 1987;225:238–46.
11. Barrack RL, Jennings RW, Wolfe MW, et al. The Coventry Award: The value of preoperative aspiration before total knee revision. Clin Orthop Rel Res 1997;345:8–16.
12. Mason JB, Fehring TK, Odum S, et al. The value of white cell count before revision total knee arthroplasty. J Arthroplasty 2003;18:1038–43.
13. Masri BA, Campbell DG, Garbuz DS, et al. Seven specialised exposures for revision hip and knee replacement. Orthop Clin North Am 1998;29:229–40.
14. Meek RMD, Greidanus NV, McGraw RW, et al. The extensile rectus snip exposure in revision of total knee arthroplasty. J Bone Joint Surg Br 2003;85–B:1120–2.
15. Toms A, Greidanus N, Garbuz D, et al. Optimally invasive exposure in revision total hip arthroplasty: a guide to selection and technique. AAOS Instructional Course Lectures. 2006;55:245–55.
16. Hubble MJW, Smith EJ. Revision of failed total hip replacement. Br J Hosp Med 1996;55(7):432–6.
17. Berry DJ, Lewallen DG, Hanssen AD, et al. Pelvic discontinuity in revision total hip arthroplasty. J Bone J Surg Am 1999;81:1692–702.
18. Quinlan JF, O'Shea K, Doyle F, et al. In-cement technique for revision hip arthroplasty. J Bone J Surg 2006;88–B:730–3.
19. Roenstein AF, MacDonald WF, Iliadis AF, et al. Revision of cemented fixation and cement-bone interface strength. Proc Inst Mech Eng (H) 1992;206:47–9.
20. Halliday BR, English HW, Timperley AJ, et al. Femoral impaction grafting with cement in revision total hip replacement. Evolution of the technique and results. J Bone J Surg Br 2003;85:809–17.
21. Kilgus DJ, Howe DJ, Strang A: Results of periprosthetic hip and knee infections caused by resistant bacteria. Clin Orthop 2002;404:116–24.

22. Trousdale RT, Hanssen AD. Infection after total knee arthroplasty. Instr Course Lect 2001;50:409–14.

23. Garvin KL, Fitzgerald RH Jr, Salvati EA, et al. Reconstruction of the infected total hip and knee arthroplasty with gentamicin-impregnated Palacos bone cement. Instr Course Lect 1993;42:293–302.

24. Mahomed NN, Barrett JA, Katz JN, et al. Rates and outcomes of primary and revision total hip replacement in the United States Medicare population. J Bone Joint Surg (Am) 2003;85–A:27–32.

25. Robinson AHN, Palmer CR, Villar RN. Is revision as good as primary hip replacement? A comparison of quality of life. J Bone Joint Surg (Br) 1999;81–B:42–5.

26. Saleh KJ, Celebrezze M, Kassim R, et al. Functional outcome after revision hip arthroplasty: a metaanalysis. Clin Orth Rel Res 2003;416:254–64.

27. Biring GS, Masri BA, Greidanus NV, et al. Predictors of quality of life outcomes after revision total hip replacement. J Bone Joint Surg 2007;89–B:1446–51.

28. Padgett DE, Kull L, Rosenburg A, et al: Revision of the acetabular component without cement after total hip arthroplasty: Three to six-year follow-up. J Bone Joint Surg (Am) 1993;75:663–73.

29. Katz RP, Dalaghan JJ, Sullivan PM, et al. Long term results of revision total hip arthroplasty using improved cementing techniques. J Bone Joint Surg (Br) 1997;79–B:322–6.

30. Lieberman JR, Moeckel BH, Evans BG, et al: Cement-within-cement revision hip arthroplasty. J Bone Joint Surg (Br) 1993;75:869–71.

31. Haddad FS, Muirhead-Allwood SK, Manktelow ARJ, et al. Two-stage uncemented revision hip arthroplasty for infection. J Bone Joint Surg Br Jul 2000;82–B:689–94.

32. Friedman RJ, Hirst P, Poss R, et al. Results of revision total knee arthroplasty performed for aseptic loosening. Clin Orthop 1990;255:235–41.

33. Hanssen AD, Rand JA. A comparison of primary and revision total knee arthroplasty using the kinematic stabiliser prosthesis. J Bone Joint Surg 1988;70A(4):491–9.

34. Wang CJ, Hsieh MC, Huang TW, et al. Clinical outcome and patient satisfaction in aseptic and septic revision total knee arthroplasty. Knee 2004;11:45–9.

35. Murray PB, Rand JA, Hanssen AD: Cemented long-stem revision total knee arthroplasty. Clin Orthop Relat Res 1994;309:116–23.

36. Whaley AL, Trousdale RT, Rand JA, et al. Cemented long-stem revision total knee arthroplasty. J Arthoplasty 2003;18:592–9.

37. Gofton WT, Tsigaras H, Butler RA, et al. Revision total knee arthroplasty: fixation with modular stems. Clin Orthop Rel Res 2002;404:158–68.

38. Fehring TK, Odum S, Olekson C, et al. Stem fixation in revision total knee replacement: a comparative analysis. Clin Orthop Rel Res 2003;416:217–24.

39. Hanssen AD, Rand JA, Osmon DR: Treatment of the infected total knee arthroplasty with insertion of another prosthesis: the effect of antibiotic-impregnated bone cement. Clin Orthop Rel Res 1994;309:44–55.

Minimally Invasive Total Hip and Knee Arthroplasty—Implications for the Elderly Patient

Inge H.F. Reininga, PhD[a,b,*], Martin Stevens, PhD[c],
Robert Wagenmakers, MD, PhD[d], Sjoerd K. Bulstra, MD, PhD[c],
Inge van den Akker-Scheek, PhD[c]

KEYWORDS

- Osteoarthritis • Older adults • Elderly • Minimally invasive surgery
- Total hip arthroplasty • Total knee arthroplasty

KEY POINTS

- Total hip arthroplasty and total knee arthroplasty have proven to be effective surgical procedures for the treatment of hip and knee osteoarthritis. In recent decades, there have been considerable efforts to further improve the component designs, modes of fixation, and surgical techniques. Minimally invasive techniques for total hip arthroplasty and total knee arthroplasty are examples of these developments.
- Minimally invasive total joint arthroplasty aims at decreasing the surgical incision and minimizing damage to the underlying soft tissue to accelerate postoperative recovery and an earlier return to normal function.

OSTEOARTHRITIS OF THE HIP AND KNEE

Osteoarthritis (OA) is one of the leading causes of musculoskeletal pain and restricted joint function worldwide, with a major negative impact on the daily physical functioning and health-related quality of life of affected patients, especially in the elderly.[1–3] Although OA may affect any joint of the body, it most commonly affects the hip and the knee. Reported prevalence rates for symptomatic OA rates of the hip in men and women age 45 years or older vary between 8.7% and 9.3%, whereas symptomatic

[a] Department of Traumatology, University of Groningen, University Medical Center Groningen, PO Box 30.001, 9700 RB Groningen, The Netherlands; [b] Department of Orthopedics, Martini Hospital Groningen, Van Swietenplein 1, 9728 NT Groningen, The Netherlands; [c] Department of Orthopedics, University of Groningen, University Medical Center Groningen, PO Box 30.001 9700 RB Groningen, The Netherlands; [d] Department of Orthopedics, Amphia Hospital Breda, Langendijk 75, 4819 EV Breda, The Netherlands
* Corresponding author. Department of Traumatology, University of Groningen, University Medical Center Groningen, PO Box 30.001, 9700 RB Groningen, The Netherlands.
E-mail address: i.h.f.reininga@umcg.nl

Clin Geriatr Med 28 (2012) 447–458
http://dx.doi.org/10.1016/j.cger.2012.05.009
0749-0690/12/$ – see front matter © 2012 Elsevier Inc. All rights reserved.
geriatric.theclinics.com

knee OA is reported to affect 13.5% of men and 18.7% of women age 45 years or older.[4] Although OA is not an inevitable consequence of aging, aging is the strongest identified risk factor for the development of the condition.[5] Another factor affecting the prevalence of OA is the growing epidemic of obesity, which is recognized as another important risk factor for OA.[6–8]

The treatment of symptomatic OA depends on the stage of the disease. Patients with mild-to-moderate OA predominantly complain of pain or stiffness of the affected joints, which hinders performance of activities of daily living mildly to moderately. Conservative treatment may be warranted for these patients. Such treatment focuses on reduction of pain and stiffness and on maintenance and improvement of functional capacities. Long-term goals are preventing progression of joint damage and improving quality of life.[9] Main conservative treatment modalities are nonpharmacologic (eg, physical therapy, education, weight reduction, braces) and pharmacologic (eg, nonsteroidal anti-inflammatory drugs, corticosteroids, hyaluronates, glucosamine, analgesics). In many patients with hip or knee OA, a combination of nonpharmacologic and pharmacologic modalities of therapy is required for an optimal and tailored management.[2,9–11] In patients with advanced hip or knee OA, total hip arthroplasty (THA) or total knee arthroplasty (TKA) have become the preferred treatment modality.[10–12]

In the past decades, considerable efforts have been made to further improve component designs, modes of fixation, and surgical techniques involved in THA and TKA. Minimally invasive techniques (MIS) for THA and TKA are examples of these developments. MIS total joint arthroplasty aims at decreasing the surgical incision and minimizing damage to the underlying soft tissue to accelerate postoperative recovery and an earlier return to normal function. The objective of this article is to report on these developments in MIS total hip and knee arthroplasty and their implications for the elderly.

TOTAL HIP AND KNEE ARTHROPLASTY

In the last century, THA and TKA have developed into very successful, reliable, and widespread treatment modalities for advanced hip and knee OA.[2] For most persons, especially for the elderly, total joint arthroplasty is a very successful surgical procedure, alleviating joint pain, restoring physical functioning, and enhancing health-related quality of life. A total of 208,600 primary THAs and 450,000 primary TKAs were performed in the United States in 2005[13] and 20,451 THAs and 20,266 TKAs in the Netherlands in 2008.[14] In the coming decades, these numbers are expected to increase dramatically. Based on demographic projections and historical trends, it is estimated that in the United States the demand for primary THAs will grow by 174% to 572,000 by 2030. The demand for primary TKAs is projected to grow by 673% to 3.48 million procedures.[13] Similar increases are expected in other Western countries.[14,15]

The increasing demand for THA and TKA is partly caused by a wider prevalence of hip and knee OA in an aging society and to the expanding indications for THA and TKA, including the elderly, who were previously considered to be too old for this kind of surgery. Research has found good clinical and functional outcomes of total joint arthroplasty in elderly patients between 65 and 75 years of age.[16–18] Additionally, several studies[18–20] have found that the oldest elderly, age 80 or older, also derive significant benefits from total joint arthroplasty, although the risk of medical complications, infection, longer hospital stay, and mortality was higher in this age group.[18]

Total Hip Arthroplasty

In the 1960s, Sir John Charnley revolutionized the surgical management of patients with osteoarthritis of the hip by introducing the concept of low-friction THA, which is now considered to be the beginning of modern total hip arthroplasty. Since then, THA has developed into one of the most successful orthopedic interventions of the last 50 years, with 10-year survival rates of implanted prostheses exceeding 90%.[21,22] From the large numbers of studies available, it can be concluded that THA results in pain relief, improves physical function, and enhances health-related quality of life, regardless of patients' characteristics, type of operation, or type of prosthesis.[23]

THA can be performed using several different approaches to the hip joint, defined by their relation to the gluteus medius muscle: anterior, anterolateral, direct lateral, transtrochanteric, and posterolateral. The posterolateral approach is the most commonly used.[24]

Modern prosthetic implants used in THA consist of an acetabular cup with a now frequently modular, articular insert, a femoral component (stem), and a modular head. There are many types of hip prostheses that differ in design and material of the cup and stem (frequently cobalt-chrome or titanium alloys) as well as composition of the articulating surfaces. So far, no component design or articulation couple has proven to be superior, although differences in survival rates exist between prostheses. The choice for a certain type of prosthesis depends on several factors, including bone quality, age, and health condition of the patient.

Fixation methods of the implant include cemented, cementless, and hybrid techniques. With the cemented technique, the implant is fixated to the bone by means of bone cement. The bone cement, an acrylic polymer called *polymethylmethacrylate*, acts as a space filler and holds the implant in position. The cementless method uses press-fit implants, which have a coated (eg, hydroxyapatite) or structured surface to encourage bone growth into the surface to hold the implant in place. Press-fit implants require solid bone for fixation; therefore, weak osteoporotic bone will tend not to tolerate a press-fit implant. Additionally, a combination of cemented and cementless techniques are used, that is, hybrid techniques. A hybrid total hip arthroplasty has one component of the implant, usually the acetabular component, inserted without bone cement, and the other component, usually the femoral component, fixated with cement.

An alternative type of hip arthroplasty, the hip resurfacing arthroplasty (HRA), has gained popularity during the last decade. The HRA procedure consists of placing a cobalt-chrome metal cap, which is hollow and shaped like a mushroom, over the head of the femur, while a matching metal cup (similar to what is used with a THR) is placed in the acetabulum, thereby replacing the articulating surfaces of the hip joint. The ideal candidate for HRA is considered to be a young active man with normal proximal femoral bone geometry and quality. Absolute contraindications include elderly patients with osteoporotic bone and impaired renal function.[25]

One of the most important factors for failure of a hip prosthesis is aseptic loosening of the prosthesis. Aseptic loosening in THA is generally caused by wear of the liner of the acetabular cup, leading to secondary osteolysis around the cup.[26,27] Hence, articular interfaces of different materials have been developed in an attempt to reduce wear. Polyethylene still remains one of the standards for bearing surfaces in joint arthroplasty. Metallic and ceramic materials are also used. The various combinations include metal-on-polyethylene, ceramic-on-polyethylene, metal-on-metal, and ceramic-on-ceramic bearings.[28]

Total Knee Arthroplasty

Total knee arthroplasty has been a standard treatment for advanced OA of the knee since the 1970s, and long-term survivorship has been reported with implant survival rates as high as 95% after 15 to 20 years.[29,30] Knee arthroplasty can be performed as a total or a partial procedure, called *unicompartmental arthroplasty*. Knee arthroplasty consists of replacing the diseased or damaged joint surfaces of the tibia and femur with metal and polyethylene implants to restore alignment and function of the knee. The knee can be divided into 3 compartments: medial (the inside part of the knee), lateral (the outside), and patellofemoral (the joint between the kneecap and the thighbone). Most patients with OA who consider knee replacement have significant wear in 2 or more of the above compartments and are best treated with a TKA. Conventional TKA is typically performed using a medial parapatellar surgical approach, which provides excellent exposure of the knee joint and offers ample room for the alignment and cutting tools used in preparing the bone for implementation of the prosthesis. A major drawback of this approach is a considerable incision of the quadriceps tendon. In addition, conventional TKA also involves lateral inversion of the patella. Both are associated with having a negative effect on the rehabilitation.[29]

Unicompartmental knee arthroplasty (UKA) is considered an option in a minority of patients whose wear is confined primarily to 1 compartment, usually the medial. Advocates of UKA cite several advantages over TKA, including a smaller incision; easier postoperative rehabilitation; better postoperative ROM; shorter hospital stay; less blood loss; lower risk of infection, stiffness, and thrombosis; and easier revision of the prosthesis if necessary.[31] Although most recent data suggest that UKA in properly selected patients has survival rates comparable with that of TKA, most surgeons believe that TKA is the more reliable long-term procedure.[32]

In knee arthroplasty, it can be decided whether the posterior cruciate ligament should be preserved or sacrificed. So far, there is no definitive answer to this issue. Long-term follow-up studies do not show any significant differences, and although it is suggested that gait function will be less abnormal if the ligament is preserved, especially when walking up and down stairs, most recent studies claim that there are no significant differences.[33] One theoretical way of incorporating normal kinematics and maximal conformity is with mobile tibial bearings. Current midterm follow-up studies of these prostheses have so far shown encouraging results.[34] The fixation method of the prosthesis is comparable with that of THA: a knee prosthesis can be fixated with cement or cementless by means of press-fit.[35] Until now, cemented total knee replacements have remained the criterion standard for TKA, but use of cementless designs with bioactive surfaces (eg, hydroxyapatite) is showing promising midterm results.[35] Finally, just as in THA, one of the most important factors for failure of the prosthesis is aseptic loosening. Aseptic loosening in TKA is generally caused by wear of the polyethylene articular surface, eventually leading to clinical failure of the prosthesis.[36]

MINIMALLY INVASIVE TOTAL JOINT ARTHROPLASTY

Although THA and TKA have proven to be highly effective surgical procedures for the treatment of hip and knee OA, there has been considerable effort in recent decades to further improve the component designs, modes of fixation, and surgical techniques.[37,38] Driven by the growing demand for total joint arthroplasty, together with a greater emphasis on cost effectiveness in health care and patients' higher expectations of shorter hospital stays and faster recovery, alternative surgical procedures have been developed aiming to further improve the success of total joint arthroplasty.

Minimally invasive (MIS) total hip and knee arthroplasty are examples of these developments. MIS total joint arthroplasty aims at decreasing the surgical incision and minimizing damage to the underlying soft tissue to accelerate postoperative recovery and an earlier return to normal function.[39,40]

Minimally Invasive Total Hip Arthroplasty

As for conventional THA, there is a wide variety of MIS THA procedures: the anterior,[41,42] anterolateral,[43,44] posterolateral,[45] posterior,[46] and posterior 2-incision[47,48] approaches. Of these, only the MIS anterior approach uses a true intermuscular plane, between the sartorius and tensor fascia latae muscles. In all of the other approaches, some degree of muscle or tendon splitting or detaching occurs as part of the surgical procedure. Hence, a critical look at the literature on MIS THA reveals that the term *minimally invasive* is often used for a conventional THA technique performed through a smaller skin incision (ie, less-invasive surgery or mini-incision THA).[49,50]

Despite the increase in use of MIS THA, its risks and benefits are still ongoing issues of debate in the orthopedic community. The different approaches for MIS THA have shown variable results,[50] which might be largely attributed to the fact that some of these so-called minimally invasive techniques, as stated before, are actually not minimally invasive. Moreover, the literature lacks well-designed studies of high methodologic quality on MIS THA.[49-51] Proponents of MIS THA claim that it results in less soft tissue trauma (smaller skin incision and less muscle damage), shorter operating time, reduced blood loss, and fewer blood transfusion requirements. Postoperative benefits include less pain, shorter hospital stay, and a quicker return to function.[52,53] The claimed benefits of a shorter operating time and reduced blood loss were confirmed in a systematic review.[49] However, only moderate evidence for a shorter length of stay was found, and the claimed benefit of a quicker return to function could not be confirmed.[49]

Opponents claim that MIS THA introduces additional risks caused by limited visibility of anatomic landmarks and vital structures.[54] Complications involve higher risks for thromboembolism, infection, neurovascular injury, femoral fracture, and component malposition, which can result in increased prosthetic wear.[55,56] Three systematic reviews reported no significant increase in perioperative complication rates after MIS THA.[49-51] The limited visibility of anatomic landmarks and vital structures during surgery is an important aspect of MIS THA that should not be ignored. The use of computer navigation during MIS THA might be the solution for the reduced visibility during surgery. Computer navigation systems not only help the surgeon with regard to the position and orientation of prosthetic components, but surgeons are also provided with instant information and feedback, allowing for more informed decision making during surgery.[57]

Minimally Invasive Total Knee Arthroplasty

In TKA, the anterior medial parapatellar approach has long been the standard approach.[29] Although there are different definitions of MIS TKA, it can be generally stated that MIS TKA involves a set of techniques for minimizing trauma to the joint and the surrounding soft tissue.[29] Hallmarks of MIS TKA include reduction of skin incision size, minimal or no incision of the extensor muscles and quadriceps tendon, minimal or no eversion of the patella, and making bone cuts in situ with minimal dislocation of the knee joint. Five approaches can be discerned that are commonly used for MIS TKA: the mini-medial parapatellar approach, the mini-midvastus approach, the mini-subvastus approach, the direct lateral approach and the quadriceps muscle-sparing approach.[58] In particular, the quadriceps-sparing (QS) approach has been developed as the least-invasive to the extensor mechanism by limiting medial parapatellar arthrotomy to the superior pole of the patella.[59] Recently, modifications of the mini-medial parapatellar, mini-subvastus, and mini-midvastus approaches applying MIS techniques have been reported and recognized as another line of MIS.[60] However, these quadriceps-sparing or modified MIS approaches have not been scientifically evaluated and compared with conventional approaches.

Proponents of MIS TKA claim benefits compared with conventional TKA in terms of less postoperative pain and faster recovery of knee function after surgery, faster rehabilitation with reduced need for assistive devices, shorter hospital stay, decreased need for stay in a skilled nursing facility during the postoperative period, and improved cosmetic appearance.[29,30,56,59,61,62] However, it must be acknowledged that these results come from prospective studies of moderate quality with short follow-up periods. Multicenter studies with longer follow-up periods are needed to justify the long-term advantages of MIS TKA over conventional TKA.[63]

Opponents of MIS TKA argue that it remains controversial whether MIS TKA is really minimally invasive and that it is associated with an increased incidence of delayed wound healing, infection, and component malaligment.[39,63–65] The minimal invasiveness of MIS TKA is questioned, because minimally invasive techniques do not necessarily reduce muscle damage, particularly in patients with an m. vastus medialis obliquus inserting at or near the midpole of the patella. Other intraoperative factors, besides minimal-skin or minimal-muscle incision, might also affect degree of muscle damage, such as ligament release, retention of the posterior cruciate ligament (PCL), tourniquet times, operating time, and blood loss.[39] Cheng and colleagues[64] concluded that although MIS TKA leads to faster recovery compared with conventional TKA, it is associated with more frequent delayed wound healing and infections. Kolisek and coworkers[65] showed that minimal-incision TKA showed no improvement over a conventional approach. There were no differences in blood loss, operating time, or early clinical and radiographic results in their study. Khanna and colleagues[63] argue in their systematic review that the benefits of MIS TKA need to be balanced against the incidence of increased tourniquet time and increased incidence of component malaligment. To that end, computer navigation systems have been developed, which might increase the accuracy of TKA. By using computer navigation during MIS TKA, accurate coronal, sagittal, and rotational component alignment may be preserved.[66]

IMPLICATIONS FOR ELDERLY THA AND TKA PATIENTS

Western society is aging. Within this growing elderly population, the group of the "oldest old" (age >80) is the fastest-growing segment.[18,67,68] Not only does the longevity of the population continue to increase, but the years of good health are increasing too, increasing the number of people aged 80 or older who are fit enough to benefit from total joint arthroplasty. As total joint arthroplasty has proven to be a reliable and successful treatment for patients with advanced OA, and the attention for health-related quality of life and maintenance of independence in the elderly population is also growing, orthopedic surgeons are increasingly willing to perform a total joint arthroplasty in this subset of the population. However, this tendency is not reflected in the mean age of patients undergoing THA or TKA, which remains more or less the same. This might be because there is also an increasing number of people who were previously considered to be too young for this procedure and who are undergoing a total joint arthroplasty. On the other hand, this may also reflect that, although orthopedic surgeons are generally more willingly to perform a TKA or a THA in the elderly, they are still reluctant to perform an arthroplasty. This might have to do less with the age of the patient than with the associated comorbidity and potential postoperative complications among elderly patients.[18,20,67]

Several studies have been conducted in which the outcomes of THA and TKA were analyzed in elderly patients (age ≥80). In a study by Clement and coworkers,[18] it was concluded that outcome after THA and TKA in patients aged 80 or older is equal to that of their younger counterparts (age 65 to 74 years), and that they are more satisfied with their prosthesis than those in the younger age group. Jones and colleagues[20] came to the same conclusion in a study in which a group of patients age 80 or older were compared with patients age 55 to 79. The older age group reported significant pain relief and functional improvement as well as positive gains in health-related quality of life that were comparable with those of the younger cohort. Additionally, they found that both groups had similar numbers of comorbid conditions and complications. Still, patients in the older age group were more likely to be transferred to a rehabilitation facility than younger patients. This, however, might be because of the social circumstances of these elderly patients (more often living alone) than a consequence of their medical condition. By contrast, Clement and colleagues[18] reported that, although the outcome after THA and TKA in patients aged 80 and older is equal to that of their younger counterparts, it was accompanied by an increased risk of medical complications, need for high dependency unit, readmission, and joint infection, leading to increased length of hospital stay and mortality. A study by Kreder and colleagues[67] assessed the risk of complications after primary THA and TKA in patients in the 80+ age group. Data from 4057 patients in that age group were compared with the results of 22,262 patients aged between 65 and 79. Patients in the older group were 3.4 times more likely to die, 2.7 times more likely to sustain a myocardial infarction, and 3.5 times more likely to get pneumonia. Postoperative confusion and urinary tract infections were also significantly more common in this older group. Hence, it can be concluded that patients age 80 and older are at a higher risk for death and serious complications after primary THA or TKA. However, Kreder and colleagues[67] argue that the overall event rate remains low, concluding that THA and TKA should continue to be offered to elderly patients, provided that the complication rates are acceptable to these patients and their families. In a study by Alfonso and coworkers[69] that evaluated the results of a group of 25 patients age 90 or older undergoing THA or TKA, it was concluded that, although the immediate postoperative course may be more difficult than in younger patients, these 90+ patients experience pain reduction and somewhat higher functional capacity compared with their preoperative status. The authors argue that THA and TKA patients in this cohort should be informed that they have a higher likelihood of experiencing perioperative medical complications and of receiving a blood transfusion than younger individuals.[69] They also argue considering inclusion of the following interventions for elderly patients: cardiac telemetry for the first 4 days after surgery, urologic prophylaxis, and the institution of environmental changes during hospitalization (eg, brighter surroundings, decreased noise levels, regular schedule) to decrease the likelihood of postoperative delirium.[69]

Based on the aforementioned studies, it can be concluded that elderly patients have an increased risk for serious complications after primary THA or TKA. Nevertheless, the overall event rate remains low. This conclusion is in line with research by Leung and coworkers[70] who infer that the postoperative mortality rate in geriatric surgical patients undergoing noncardiac surgery is low. Illustrative in this respect are the findings of Alfonso and colleagues[69] that the survival rates of patients who had undergone THA or TKA were greater than those of age-matched controls, a seemingly paradoxical result that is probably due to a selection bias: a patient age 90 or older who is selected to undergo total joint arthroplasty is more likely to be healthier than the average individual of the same age. Berend and colleagues[71] and Clement and colleagues[18] found similar results among the extremely elderly undergoing THA or TKA. Overall, it can be concluded that THA and TKA are appropriate options for patients fit enough to endure surgery, irrespective of their age. With increasing life expectancy and elective surgery improving the quality of life, age is not the only factor that affects the outcome of a THA, and TKA and should not be the limiting factor when deciding whether to perform surgery.

Little research has been conducted so far on the implications of MIS THA and MIS TKA in elderly patients. To our knowledge, only one study has explored the implications of minimally invasive total joint arthroplasty in the elderly. Müller and coworkers[72] investigated the consequences of minimally invasive THA compared with conventional THA in a group of elderly patients (age >70), then compared the results with those of a group of younger patients (age <70). The results of that study showed an age-related impact on clinical outcome after THA. The researchers argue that the rationale for the poorer functional outcome after THA in the elderly seems to be substantiated by muscular changes. The skeletal musculature of elderly patients possesses a higher vulnerability and a reduced regenerative capacity. Moreover, elderly patients are characterized by a higher incidence of postoperative fatty muscle atrophy, which is associated with reduced muscular function. However, more important is the finding that older patients who underwent THA through a conventional approach had a significantly higher grade of muscle atrophy than older patients who underwent a minimally invasive approach. This approach-dependent effect was not evident in the younger patient group, which obviously possesses a sufficient regenerative capacity. It seems that the musculature of younger patients is able to compensate better after a more invasive surgical approach; hence, the potential benefits of an MIS approach do not become evident. By contrast, Müller and colleagues[72] conclude that clear structural differences are noticeable in elderly patients, who noticeably seem to benefit from a minimally invasive approach. So far, results with respect to MIS TKA are lacking. However, it can be hypothesized that the potential benefits of an MIS approach reported in THA also are applicable to MIS TKA.

SUMMARY

Overall, it can be concluded that because of the aging society, an increasing number of elderly people will be undergoing total joint arthroplasty. These elderly patients have an increased risk for serious complications after primary THA or TKA. However, the overall complication rates remain low. The use of MIS total joint arthroplasty is also increasing, although its risks and benefits are still an ongoing issue of debate in the orthopedic community. MIS total joint arthroplasty aims at decreasing the surgical incision and minimizing damage to the underlying soft tissue to accelerate postoperative recovery and an earlier return to normal function. A critical look at the literature on MIS shows that the term *minimally invasive* is often used for a conventional total joint arthroplasty performed through a smaller skin incision. Research has shown promising results of using MIS in elderly patients; it seems that compared with younger patients, elderly patients benefit more from a minimally invasive approach.

REFERENCES

1. Dekker J, Boot B, van der Woude LH, et al. Pain and disability in osteoarthritis: a review of biobehavioral mechanisms. J Behav Med 1992;15(2):189–214.
2. Felson DT, Lawrence RC, Dieppe PA, et al. Osteoarthritis: new insights. Part 1: the disease and its risk factors. Ann Intern Med 2000;133(8):635–46.

3. Guccione AA, Felson DT, Anderson JJ. Defining arthritis and measuring functional status in elders: methodological issues in the study of disease and physical disability. Am J Public Health 1990;80(8):945–9.

4. Lawrence RC, Felson DT, Helmick CG, et al. Estimates of the prevalence of arthritis and other rheumatic conditions in the United States: Part II. Arthritis & Rheumatism 2008;58(1):26–35.

5. Sharma L, Kapoor D, Issa S. Epidemiology of osteoarthritis: an update. Curr Opin Rheumatol 2006;18(2):147–56.

6. Holliday KL, McWilliams DF, Maciewicz RA, et al. Lifetime body mass index, other anthropometric measures of obesity and risk of knee or hip osteoarthritis in the GOAL case-control study. Osteoarthritis Cartilage 2011;19(1):37–43.

7. Cooper C, Snow S, McAlindon TE, et al. Risk factors for the incidence and progression of radiographic knee osteoarthritis. Arthritis Rheum 2000;43(5):995–1000.

8. Apold H, Meyer HE, Espehaug B, et al. Weight gain and the risk of total hip replacement a population-based prospective cohort study of 265,725 individuals. Osteoarthritis Cartilage 2011;19(7):809–15.

9. Bijlsma JW, Berenbaum F, Lafeber FP. Osteoarthritis: an update with relevance for clinical practice. Lancet 2011;377(9783):2115–26.

10. Zhang W, Moskowitz RW, Nuki G, et al. OARSI recommendations for the management of hip and knee osteoarthritis, Part II: OARSI evidence-based, expert consensus guidelines. Osteoarthritis Cartilage 2008;16(2):137–62.

11. Zhang W, Doherty M. EULAR recommendations for knee and hip osteoarthritis: a critique of the methodology. Br J Sports Med 2006;40(8):664–9.

12. Zhang W, Moskowitz RW, Nuki G, et al. OARSI recommendations for the management of hip and knee osteoarthritis, part I: critical appraisal of existing treatment guidelines and systematic review of current research evidence. Osteoarthritis Cartilage 2007;15(9):981–1000.

13. Kurtz S, Ong K, Lau E, et al. Projections of primary and revision hip and knee arthroplasty in the United States from 2005 to 2030. J Bone Joint Surg Am 2007; 89(4):780–5.

14. Otten R, van Roermund PM, Picavet HS. Trends in the number of knee and hip arthroplasties: considerably more knee and hip prostheses due to osteoarthritis in 2030. Ned Tijdschr Geneeskd 2010;154:A1534.

15. Pedersen AB, Johnsen SP, Overgaard S, et al. Total hip arthroplasty in Denmark: incidence of primary operations and revisions during 1996–2002 and estimated future demands. Acta Orthop 2005;76(2):182–9.

16. Hamel MB, Toth M, Legedza A, et al. Joint replacement surgery in elderly patients with severe osteoarthritis of the hip or knee: decision making, postoperative recovery, and clinical outcomes. Arch Intern Med 2008;168(13):1430–40.

17. Nilsdotter AK, Lohmander LS. Age and waiting time as predictors of outcome after total hip replacement for osteoarthritis. Rheumatology (Oxford) 2002;41(11):1261–7.

18. Clement ND, MacDonald D, Howie CR, et al. The outcome of primary total hip and knee arthroplasty in patients aged 80 years or more. J Bone Joint Surg (Br) 2011; 93B(9):1265–70.

19. Birdsall PD, Hayes JH, Cleary R, et al. Health outcome after total knee replacement in the very elderly. J Bone Joint Surg Br 1999;81(4):660–2.

20. Jones C, Voaklander D, Johnston W, et al. The effect of age on pain, function, and quality of life after total hip and knee arthroplasty. Arch Intern Med 2001;161(3): 454–60.

21. Callaghan JJ, Albright JC, Goetz DD, et al. Charnley total hip arthroplasty with cement. Minimum twenty-five-year follow-up. J Bone Joint Surg Am 2000;82(4): 487–97.
22. Havelin LI, Engesaeter LB, Espehaug B, et al. The Norwegian Arthroplasty Register: 11 years and 73,000 arthroplasties. Acta Orthop Scand 2000;71(4):337–53.
23. Montin L, Leino-Kilpi H, Suominen T, et al. A systematic review of empirical studies between 1966 and 2005 of patient outcomes of total hip arthroplasty and related factors. J Clin Nurs 2008;17(1):40–5.
24. Kelmanovich D, Parks ML, Sinha R, et al. Surgical approaches to total hip arthroplasty. J South Orthop Assoc 2003;12(2):90–4.
25. Shimmin AJ. Complications associated with hip resurfacing arthroplasty. Orthop Clin North Am 2005;36(2):187–93.
26. Sochart DH. Relationship of acetabular wear to osteolysis and loosening in total hip arthroplasty. Clin Orthop Relat Res 1999;(363)(363):135–50.
27. Learmonth ID, Young C, Rorabeck C. The operation of the century: total hip replacement. Lancet 2007;370(9597):1508–19.
28. Lee K, Goodman SB. Current state and future of joint replacements in the hip and knee. Exp Rev Med Device 2008;5(3):383–93.
29. Mont MA, Zywiel MG, McGrath MS, et al. Scientific evidence for minimally invasive total knee arthroplasty. Instr Course Lect 2010;59:73–82.
30. Watanabe T, Muneta T, Ishizuki M. Is a minimally invasive approach superior to a conventional approach for total knee arthroplasty? Early outcome and 2-to 4-year follow-up. J Orthopaed Sci 2009;14(5):589–95.
31. Saccomanni B. Unicompartmental knee arthroplasty: a review of literature. Clin Rheumatol 2010;29(4):339–46.
32. McAllister CM. The role of unicompartmental knee arthroplasty versus total knee arthroplasty in providing maximal performance and satisfaction. J Knee Surg 2008; 21(4):286–92.
33. Joglekar S, Gioe TJ, Yoon P, et al. Gait analysis comparison of cruciate retaining and substituting TKA following PCL sacrifice. Knee 2011.
34. Callaghan JJ. Mobile-bearing knee replacement: clinical results: a review of the literature. Clin Orthop Relat Res 2001;(392)(392):221–5.
35. Meneghini RM, Hanssen AD. Cementless fixation in total knee arthroplasty: past, present, and future. J Knee Surg 2008;21(4):307–14.
36. Schmalzried T, Callaghan J. Wear in total hip and knee replacements. J Bone Joint Surg Am 1999;81A(1):115–36.
37. Laskin RS. Minimally invasive total knee arthroplasty—The results justify its use. Clin Orthop 2005;(440):54–9.
38. Dennis DA. Trends in total knee arthroplasty. Orthopedics 2006;29(9 Suppl):S13–6.
39. Niki Y, Mochizuki T, Momohara S, et al. Is minimally invasive surgery in total knee arthroplasty really minimally invasive surgery? J Arthroplasty 2009;24(4):499–504.
40. Berend KR, Lombardi AV Jr, Seng BE, et al. Enhanced early outcomes with the anterior supine intermuscular approach in primary total hip arthroplasty. J Bone Joint Surg Am 2009;91 (Suppl 6):107–20.
41. Matta JM, Shahrdar C, Ferguson T. Single-incision anterior approach for total hip arthroplasty on an orthopaedic table. Clin Orthop Relat Res 2005;441:115–24.
42. Rachbauer F. Minimally invasive total hip arthroplasty via direct anterior approach. Orthopade 2005;34(11):1106–8.
43. Bertin KC, Rottinger H. Anterolateral mini-incision hip replacement surgery: a modified Watson-Jones approach. Clin Orthop Relat Res 2004;(429):248–55.

44. Martin R, Clayson PE, Troussel S, et al. Anterolateral minimally invasive total hip arthroplasty. a prospective randomized controlled study with a follow-up of 1 year. J Arthroplasty 2011;26(8):1362–72.
45. Young-Hoo K. Comparison of primary total hip arthroplasties performed with a minimally invasive technique or a standard technique: a prospective and randomized study. J Arthroplasty 2006;21(8):1092–8.
46. Dorr LD, Maheshwari AV, Long WT, et al. Early pain relief and function after posterior minimally invasive and conventional total hip arthroplasty. A prospective, randomized, blinded study. J Bone Joint Surg Am 2007;89(6):1153–60.
47. Berger RA. The technique of minimally invasive total hip arthroplasty using the two-incision approach. Instr Course Lect 2004;53:149–55.
48. Duwelius PJ, Burkhart RL, Hayhurst JO, et al. Comparison of the 2-incision and mini-incision posterior total hip arthroplasty technique: a retrospective match-pair controlled study. J Arthroplasty 2007;22(1):48–56.
49. Reininga IHF, Zijlstra W, Wagenmakers R, et al. Minimally invasive and computer-navigated total hip arthroplasty: a qualitative and systematic review of the literature. BMC Musculoskeletal Disorders 2010;11:92.
50. Cheng T, Feng JG, Liu T, et al. Minimally invasive total hip arthroplasty: a systematic review. Int Orthop 2009;33(6):1473–81.
51. Smith TO, Blake V, Hing CB. Minimally invasive versus conventional exposure for total hip arthroplasty: a systematic review and meta-analysis of clinical and radiological outcomes. Int Orthop 2011;35(2):173–84.
52. Chimento GF, Pavone V, Sharrock N, et al. Minimally invasive total hip arthroplasty: a prospective randomized study. J Arthroplasty 2005;20(2):139–44.
53. Howell JR, Masri BA, Duncan CP. Minimally invasive versus standard incision antero-lateral hip replacement: a comparative study. Orthop Clin North Am 2004;35:153–62.
54. Callaghan J. Skeptical perspectives on minimally invasive total hip arthroplasty. J Bone Joint Surg Am 2006;85 A:2242–3.
55. Pagnano MW, Leone J, Lewallen DG, et al. Two-incision THA had modest outcomes and some substantial complications. Clin Orthop Relat Res 2005;441:86–90.
56. Woolson ST, Mow CS, Syquia JF, et al. Comparison of primary total hip replacements performed with a standard incision or a mini-incision. J Bone Joint Surg Am 2004; 86–A(7):1353–8.
57. DiGioia AM, Hafez MA. "MIS meets CAOS"—less and minimally invasive joint recon-struction. Int J Med Robot Comput Assist Surg 2005;1(4):6–7.
58. Bonutti PM, Zywiel MG, McGrath MS, et al. Surgical techniques for minimally invasive exposures for total knee arthroplasty. Instr Course Lect 2010;59:83–91.
59. Tria AJ, Coon TM. Minimal incision total knee arthroplasty—Early experience. Clin Orthop 2003;(416):185–90.
60. Scuderi G, Tenholder M, Capeci C. Surgical approaches in mini-incision total knee arthroplasty. Clin Orthop 2004;(428):61–7.
61. Bonutti PM, Mont MA, McMahon M, et al. Minimally invasive total knee arthroplasty. J Bone Joint Surgery Am 2004;86A:26–32.
62. Laskin R, Beksac B, Phongjunakorn A, et al. Minimally invasive total knee replacement through a mini-midvastus incision—An outcome study. Clin Orthop 2004;(428):74–81.
63. Khanna A, Gougoulias N, Longo UG, et al. Minimally invasive total knee arthroplasty: a systematic review. Orthop Clin North Am 2009;40(4):479.
64. Cheng T, Liu T, Zhang G, et al. Does minimally invasive surgery improve short-term recovery in total knee arthroplasty? Clin Orthop 2010;468(6):1635–48.

65. Kolisek FR, Bonutti PM, Hozack WJ, et al. Clinical experience using a minimally invasive surgical approach for total knee arthroplasty— early results of a prospective randomized study compared to a standard approach. J Arthroplasty 2007; 22(1):8–13.

66. Biasca N, Wirth S, Bungartz M. Mechanical accuracy of navigated minimally invasive total knee arthroplasty (MIS TKA). Knee 2009;16(1):22–9.

67. Kreder H, Berry G, McMurtry I, et al. Arthroplasty in the octogenarian— quantifying the risks. J Arthroplasty 2005;20(3):289–93.

68. Population prognosis 2010–2060: increased population aging, longer life span. Available at: http://www.cbs.nl/NR/rdonlyres/91E3EC1E-4FF2-4019-B47E24DC24334180/0/2010bevolkingsprognose20102060sterkerevergrijzingart.pdf. Accessed December 12, 2011.

69. Alfonso DT, Howell D, Strauss EJ, et al. Total hip and knee arthroplasty in nonagenarians. J Arthroplasty 2007;22(6):807–11.

70. Leung J, Dzankic S. Relative importance of preoperative health status versus intraoperative factors in predicting postoperative adverse outcomes in geriatric surgical patients. J Am Geriatr Soc 2001;49(8):1080–5.

71. Berend M, Thong A, Faris G, et al. Total joint arthroplasty in the extremely elderly—Hip and knee arthroplasty after entering the 89th year of life. J Arthroplasty 2003;18(7): 817–21.

72. Müller M, Tohtz S, Dewey M, et al. Age-related appearance of muscle trauma in primary total hip arthroplasty and the benefit of a minimally invasive approach for patients older than 70 years. Int Orthop 2011;35(2):165–71.

Pharmacologic Pain Management Before and After Total Joint Replacement of the Hip and Knee

James V. Bono, MD[a],*, Claire E. Robbins, DPT[b], Abdel K. Mehio, MD[c], Mehran Aghazadeh, MD[b], Carl T. Talmo, MD[a]

KEYWORDS

- Pain management • Older adults • Total knee replacement
- Total hip arthroplasty

KEY POINTS

- There are many effective treatment measures for osteoarthritis of the hip and knee with varying degrees of effectiveness. Nonoperative measures include patient education, physical therapy, activity modification, weight loss, and medications.
- Pharmacologic strategies include acetaminophen, nonsteroidal antiinflammatory agents, injections of cortisone or viscosupplementation, and, less commonly, tramadol or other pain relievers. In patients who may be candidates for total joint replacement, narcotic medications should be avoided to preserve their benefits for the postoperative period.
- Over the past 20 years, multimodal pain management has been beneficial to the patient undergoing total joint replacement surgery. Studies have shown this form of pain management decreases postoperative opioid consumption and the related adverse effects. Research is warranted in the areas of postoperative pain scores and patient satisfaction as institutional multimodal protocols continue to evolve.

Total knee replacement (TKR) and total hip replacement (THR) can provide pain relief and restoration of function in individuals with musculoskeletal impairment. The procedures are extremely successful and essentially unrivaled in the treatment of osteoarthritis (OA) pain. During the next few decades, the demand for total joint

Disclosure: The authors did not receive any outside funding or grants in support of their research for or preparation of this work.
[a] New England Baptist Hospital, Tufts University School of Medicine, Boston, MA, USA; [b] New England Baptist Hospital, Boston, MA, USA; [c] New England Baptist Hospital, Boston University School of Medicine, Boston, MA, USA
* Corresponding author. New England Baptist Hospital, 125 Parker Hill Avenue, Boston, MA 02120.
E-mail address: jbono@caregroup.harvard.edu

replacement in the United States is expected to increase significantly, possibly reaching near epidemic proportions. By the year 2030, it is expected that the number of THRs performed will increase by 174% and the number of TKRs could reach close to 3.48 million procedures.[1,2] Because of these factors, a detailed understanding of perioperative issues in THR and TKR is of paramount importance to all practitioners.

Total joint replacement (TJR) is one of the most successful surgical procedures today due in part to evolutionary changes in surgical technique, implants, improved patient care pathways, and pain management. A truly successful and effective procedure is achieved by developing an individual care plan that addresses pain management perioperatively. Failure to provide adequate analgesia may contribute to slower rehabilitation, joint stiffness, depression, poor patient satisfaction, increased risk of postoperative complications, and prolonged hospital stay.[3] Safe and effective pain management for the older or aging adult undergoing TJR can present a clinical challenge for the health care team. Many older patients present to the surgeon with a history of taking over-the-counter medications for pain or other prescriptions for a number of comorbidities. In addition, they may present with preexisting functional and cognitive impairments and balance issues. Therefore, clinicians need to have a keen understanding of the aging process and the associated pharmacokinetics and pharmacodynamics of the analgesics given and the potential for adverse drug reactions.

It has been almost two decades since Kehlet and Dahl[4] introduced and encouraged the use of multimodal pain management over the more traditional intravenous patient-controlled analgesia (PCA) or epidural analgesia for postoperative pain control. The principle of multimodal pain management is to use multiple agents along the pain pathway in an effort to provide adequate pain relief while reducing the use of opioids and their associated side effects. Perioperative pain management protocols using multimodal pain management in association with effective TJR surgery have been very successful at minimizing narcotic intake and the associated side effects while promoting early rehabilitation and improved patient satisfaction.

PREOPERATIVE PAIN MANAGEMENT

A primary goal of treating aging patients with OA is achieving a level of pain control that will grant them adequate function and mobility to perform activities of daily living and improve quality of life, while avoiding potential harm such as the toxicity and side effects associated with some pharmacologic agents. Many patients have exhausted nonpharmacologic resources by the time they develop moderate to severe OA of the hip or knee, and prior to considering TJR.

Initial treatment of early knee OA includes activity modification, patient education, weight loss in obese individuals, and assistive ambulatory aids such as a cane. There is reasonably good evidence that these measures will benefit patients, particularly patient education and weight loss when appropriate. Physical therapy for quadriceps strengthening and water exercises is also beneficial.[5] Treatment options for hip OA are similar; however, physical therapy and other nonoperative measures may have more limited benefit. Many guidelines have been developed regarding initial therapies for the treatment of OA of the hip and knee.[6,7] A consensus on these issues remains elusive.

As an adjunct to these measures, a number of pharmacologic agents have shown efficacy in the management of OA and also in treating patients in the preoperative period prior to TJR.

Acetaminophen

For older adults with mild to moderate musculoskeletal pain, acetaminophen is generally considered first line treatment and is the most commonly used analgesic.[8] For a large number of patients awaiting surgery, this drug is a safe and effective form of analgesia. Although the drug also has antipyretic properties, it does not have antiinflammatory activity. However, for individuals with liver or kidney disease or for those patients who consume a moderate amount of alcohol, extreme caution should be used when prescribing this drug to avoid liver or kidney toxicity. A maximum daily dose of less than 4 g is recommended.[9] Hepatotoxicity with this medication has been well-publicized and can be irreversible. Individuals taking more than 2 ounces of alcohol daily should decrease their intake of acetaminophen to less than 2 to 2.5 g per 24-hour period.

Chronic use of acetaminophen can also induce interstitial kidney disease leading to chronic renal failure, although this occurrence is believed to be relatively rare.[10] There is also some evidence of potential cardiovascular risk associated with the use of acetaminophen. Chan and colleagues[11] report that use of acetaminophen or non-steroidal antiinflammatory drugs (NSAIDs) at high frequency or dose is associated with a significant increased risk for cardiovascular events.[11]

Bradley and colleagues[12] demonstrated significant improvement in arthritis pain relief with 1000 mg of acetaminophen four times a day with effects equal to ibuprofen at lower does (1200 to 2400 mg/d), and acetaminophen was better tolerated than any dose of ibuprofen. Ibuprofen was found to provide the additional benefit of decreased rest pain when taken in the antiinflammatory dose of 2400 mg per day when compared with acetaminophen.[12]

Although diclofenac, misoprostol, and celecoxib provided better pain relief and Western Ontario and McMasters University Arthritis Index scores in a study by Pincus and colleagues,[13] acetaminophen was better tolerated with far fewer gastrointestinal (GI) side effects than either of the other medications.

In general, acetaminophen is well-tolerated with few side effects and good efficacy in OA. This low risk-to-benefit ratio makes it an excellent first line agent for patients with mild to moderate OA who are under the care of a physician.

Nonsteroidal Antiinflammatory Drugs

NSAIDs are extremely popular in the management of OA of the hip and knee. Over-the-counter availability make these medications a very convenient and accessible form of pain relief for appropriate patients, whether prescribed by a physician or not The combination of pain relieving and antiinflammatory properties as well as the ease of access make NSAIDs the most popular class of drugs used by individuals with OA.

Traditional or "nonselective" NSAIDs inhibit both cyclooxygenase-1 (COX-1) and cyclooxygenase-2 (COX-2) enzymes. COX-1 is present in most tissues and maintains the normal lining of the stomach in the GI tract. COX-2 is primarily found at the site of inflammation.[14] COX-2 inhibitors were originally developed to lower the potential lower risk of GI adverse effects such as ulcer formation, gastritis, and GI bleeding. However, the advantage of COX-2 inhibitors over traditional NSAIDs remains controversial.[14]

NSAIDs are appropriate to use in the older patient on a short-term basis with cautious and careful observation by a physician. Individual medical history, comorbidities, and concomitant medications should be carefully reviewed and discussed with the patient.

Use of NSAIDs is associated with significant morbidity and occasional toxicity in the elderly population, most notably a significant rate of bleeding and peptic ulcer disease, and therefore must be monitored closely.[8] Patients at risk for NSAID-associated side effects are candidates for earlier referral and consideration for TJR.[8,15,16] COX-2 inhibitors may be a better option in the treatment of OA for patients with a history of GI upset or bleeding.

Topical NSAIDs

Short-term use of topical NSAIDs, diclofenac sodium 1% gel and diclofenac sodium 1.5% in 45.5% dimethylsulfoxide solution, have shown safety and efficacy in treatment of knee OA pain. Absorption of topical NSAIDs may be influenced by mode of application (ultrasound, iontophoresis, or hand application) and bonding properties of the solution.[17,18] For the older adult at risk for systemic toxicity from oral NSAIDs, topical agents may offer localized pain relief, increased knee range of motion, and improved physical function prior to surgery.

Although not an NSAID, capsaicin, which is derived from pepper, has shown some benefit in clinical trials when applied as a cream or ointment four times a day. The medication can be irritating when coming into contact with mucous membranes, and care should be taken when this medication is applied.[19]

Opioids

Nonnarcotic and narcotic opioid analgesics may be prescribed for short-term use for patients with moderate to severe pain awaiting total joint replacement surgery. A commonly used nonnarcotic analgesic is tramadol, which can depress the central nervous system (CNS) and may require dose adjustment for patients with renal impairment. Tramadol may also alter the seizure threshold.[20] Side effects may include nausea, vomiting, drowsiness, and constipation.

Narcotic agents, although effective in relieving severe musculoskeletal pain, must be carefully considered prior to use with the older patient. Narcotic opioids with acetaminophen should be used cautiously to avoid toxicity. Adverse reactions of CNS depression, nausea and vomiting, or constipation may require adjuvant drugs such as antiemetics or laxatives. Also, opioid use may impair judgment or motor skills, resulting in changes in balance or falls.

Recent reports in the literature indicate chronic opioid use prior to TKR may put patients at greater risk for complications and difficulty with pain control postoperatively compared with patients who did not use opioids preoperatively.[21]

Tramadol

Although commonly used in multimodal protocols for postoperative pain management, tramadol has been successfully used in patients experiencing moderate to severe preoperative pain.[22] Tramadol should be considered for patients receiving minimal relief from acetaminophen, NSAIDs, or COX-2 selective therapy or with contraindications to other drugs.[19,22,23]

Tramadol is a nonnarcotic opioid agent that is structurally related to codeine and morphine. A centrally acting analgesic, it binds to opioid receptors and blocks the reuptake of both serotonin and norepinephrine.[24,25] It is often used in combination with acetaminophen, providing optimal analgesic benefit for acute pain.

Efficacy of tramadol is not strongly supported in all patient cohorts. It is contraindicated in patients on some antidepressant medications and those at risk for seizure. Cautionary measures should be taken with some older patients because of possible

CNS depression. Also, dose adjustment may be necessary for patients with a history of renal or liver impairment.

Tramadol is not without risk, but popularity of the drug may be attributed in part to a lower incidence of adverse effects compared with other opioids. To decrease the side effects of nausea and vomiting it is suggested to initiate therapy with a low starting dose.[23,25,26]

Intraarticular Corticosteroid Injections

Although controversial in the past, corticosteroid injections have been used for years to treat pain and inflammation of arthritic joints. The mechanism of action of corticosteroids in OA remains largely unknown. Corticosteroids have been shown to reduce prostaglandin synthesis, decrease enzymatic activity including collagenase and proteases, and also reduce inflammatory mediators such as interleukin-1 and tumor necrosis factor–alpha.[27] In addition, there is evidence of absorption into the circulation that may vary with the dose of steroid administered, and some degree of systemic effects cannot be ruled out as a potential mechanism of action for intraarticular administration of steroids.[28] This effect should also be kept in mind when administering steroids to diabetic patients who may notice an increase in blood sugars for several days following injection. These patients may need to avoid bilateral injections or multiple injections in a short period to prevent complications related to hyperglycemia.

Many studies have demonstrated decreased pain and some degree of improved function following injection; however, the magnitude and duration of the benefit is quite variable. Dieppe and colleagues[29] performed a controlled trial of triamcinolone versus placebo in 48 patients and demonstrated significant reduced pain and tenderness when compared with placebo. Other randomized studies have demonstrated benefit for steroid injection with some variability in the degree and duration of the effectiveness based on the preparation and dosage of drug administered.[30] Based on these data, triamcinolone may offer superior results over other preparations of steroid.[31] Other controlled trials have shown minimal to no benefit with repeated injections, and therefore the exact role of corticosteroid injection in the management of OA remains controversial.[32] Whereas these injections often provide short-term benefit, they do not alter the natural history of the disease, which remains progressive over time. For patients with chronic OA of the knee, the risks related to intraarticular cortisone injection are low with an extremely low rate of infection hemorrhagic effusion, transient synovitis, or hyperglycemia.[33]

In contrast, corticosteroid injections in the hip joint are reserved mainly for diagnostic purposes and have little or no role in the treatment of chronic hip OA because of a higher associated risk of infection and a higher risk of disease progression with repeated injections.[34] In addition, repeated intraarticular hip injections have demonstrated very limited benefit and no alteration in the natural history of the disease and need for THR.[35,36] Patients should be counseled on the potential risk of infection and the possibility of further bony destruction to the joint prior to seeking this type of treatment.

Viscosupplementation/Joint Fluid Therapy

Hyaluronic acid is a normal component of synovial fluid that is believed to contribute to its role in joint lubrication and mechanics. This molecule is found to have an altered chemical structure and a lowered density in the synovial fluid extracted from arthritic joints, and therefore it has been hypothesized that replenishing the arthritic knee with hyaluronic acid might provide symptomatic relief of the osteoarthritic knee.[37]

Based on these and other scientific principles, a number of commercially available preparations of hyaluronan have been tested and used in the treatment of OA of the knee. These preparations generally require anywhere from one to five injections for a single course of treatment. A number of clinical studies have demonstrated a variable degree of modest improvement in OA pain and function following intraarticular administration of these compounds.[38–40] For example, a thorough Cochrane review of the literature demonstrated an 11% to 54% improvement in pain for a 6-week period following the injections and a 9% to 15% improvement in function during that interval.[38] In general, the effects are believed to be more pronounced in patients with mild or moderate OA.[15,41] Use of hyaluronan injections in patients with severe OA is generally not recommended.

There is limited evidence available to suggest that repeated courses of treatment are advisable, and the preparations are currently not recommended in the treatment of hip disease, also because of a lack of available evidence. There is also no evidence that these preparations alter the natural history or progression of OA or lower the potential need for TJR. The medications are also not advised in patients allergic to fowl products because of the presence of rooster comb in some of the preparations. The risks related to administration are low overall; however, the incidence of transient painful synovitis and effusion seems to be higher than that seen following cortisone injection.[42,43]

MULTIMODAL PAIN MANAGEMENT
Preemptive Analgesia

Current trends in TJR pain management suggest using the concept of preemptive analgesia in combination with multimodal analgesia to achieve optimal postoperative pain management.[3,24,44]

A preemptive protocol generally includes the use analgesics and/or a combination of analgesics and antiinflammatory agents administered to the patient on the day of surgery or the day before. The concept is to block the transmission of noxious efferent information from the patient's peripheral nervous system to the spinal cord and the brain by limiting sensitization of the nervous system to painful stimuli. Therefore, dosage and timing are important. The dosage must be adequate to limit sensitization and given prior to the initial incision.[45]

An example of a preemptive analgesia protocol is shown in **Table 1**.

Preoperative Nerve Blocks

Regional anesthesia including the use of peripheral nerve blocks plays a significant role in pain management following contemporary TJR, particular TKR. Following TKR, use of oral and intravenous pain medication is complimented by use of a femoral nerve blockade. This anesthesia may be performed by a one-time injection around the femoral nerve or by continuous infusion with an indwelling femoral nerve catheter. Both methods have been shown to be effective in controlling postoperative pain with low risk and rare complications.[46,47] Indwelling catheters are placed under ultrasound guidance in the preoperative holding area on the day of surgery and have the advantage of providing anesthesia over the anterior knee for up to 48 hours postoperatively. The catheter typically remains in place for 24 hours with an infusion of .0625% bupivacaine at 3 cc/h. Single shot blockades are also effective but have a shorter duration of action, typically lasting no more than 12 hours.

Sensory innervation to the posterior aspect of the knee is provided by the sciatic nerve, and therefore posterior knee pain is not alleviated by femoral nerve blockade and requires other sources of pain control. Risks associated with regional nerve block

---

Table 1
Preoperative analgesic protocols

- **Patients less than 70 years old:**
  - ○ OxyContin 10 mg, one tablet PO once
  - ○ Acetaminophen (Tylenol) 325 mg/tab, three tabs (975 mg) PO once
  - ○ Celebrex (celecoxib) 200 mg/capsule, one capsule PO once (avoid if CR >1.3 or sulfa allergy)
- **If sulfa allergy:**
  - ○ Meloxicam (Mobic) 7.5 mg/tablet, one tablet PO once
- **Patients over 70 years old:**
  - ○ Tylenol #3, one tablet PO once
  - ○ Celebrex (celecoxib) 200 mg/capsule, one capsule PO once (avoid if CR >1.3 or sulfa allergy)
- **If sulfa allergy:**
  - ○ Meloxicam (Mobic) 7.5 mg/tablet, one tablet PO once
- For chronic pain patients (on a daily opioid for <1 month) order in addition
  - ○ Lyrica (pregabalin) 50 mg/capsule, one capsule PO once

Abbreviations: CR, creatinine level in the blood; PO, by mouth.

---

are exceedingly rare.[47] Because it is impossible to block only the sensory fibers of the nerve, motor blockade also occurs while the block is active, resulting in quadriceps weakness and the risk of falling with unsupervised ambulation. To prevent this possibility, all patients are discouraged from getting out of bed without a nurse or therapist, and patients are required to use a knee immobilizer while the block is functioning postoperatively. Patient falls represent the most common risk related to femoral nerve blockade, and therefore extreme caution must be considered when offering this modality to potentially noncompliant patients or those suffering from delirium.

Although safe and frequently used in TJR surgery, femoral nerve blocks are technically challenging and require a skilled and experienced pain management team to ensure success and avoid other potential risks such as nerve or vascular injury during insertion.[47]

The addition of preoperative femoral nerve blocks with continuous infusion to a multimodal pain management program may be beneficial in comparison with more traditional pain management techniques. At the authors' institution, femoral nerve blocks have decreased the amount of anesthetic used with general anesthesia as well as provided improved participation in postoperative range of motion protocols, better range of motion, and a lowered rate of subsequent interventions for the treatment of stiffness. In addition, with the use of regional blocks, many older patients require lowered amounts of narcotics, which may contribute to a lowered incidence of postoperative cognitive impairment.

Operative Anesthesia

Successful TJR surgery may be performed with both general and spinal anesthesia.[48,49] Spinal anesthesia is occasionally preferred for patients with cardiopulmonary comorbidities who are able to tolerate brief episodes of hypotension that frequently occur with the sympathetic blockade accompanying spinal anesthesia Historically, a combined spinal and epidural anesthesia was believed to have a high safety profile, with lowered incidence of postoperative nausea and a potentially lowered rate of deep vein thrombosis.[49] More recently, however, epidural anesthesia has been associated with a higher rate of postoperative nerve palsy and a very rare risk of epidural hematoma with modern postoperative deep vein thrombosis prophylaxis regimens, and therefore has become far less common.[50–52]

Modern general anesthesia, which is considered extremely safe, has the advantage of being very reliable and highly modifiable in all patients, and therefore has become the most common anesthetic used in TJR. The most common complication following general anesthesia is nausea, which can be easily treated with antiemetics, anesthetic agents such as midazolam and ketamine, and, rarely, with preoperative steroid administration. Additionally, a nitrous oxide anesthesia gas mixture may also be helpful for patients with a history of chronic pain.

Intraoperative Injections

Patients undergoing TKR often complain of posterior knee pain in the immediate postoperative period, particularly when femoral nerve blockade effectively diminishes anterior knee pain. To help alleviate joint pain following TKR, combinations of medications including local anesthetics, opiates, steroids, and antiinflammatories are injected into the periarticular soft tissues, with a number of different investigators reporting pain relief and decreased use of narcotic pain medications in the perioperative period.[53] Local anesthetic with epinephrine is carefully injected into the synovium, joint capsule, periosteum, and ligamentous structures, with the added potential benefit of providing vasoconstriction of small vessels in these tissues and potentially reduced bleeding. The authors prefer an injection of bupivacaine with epinephrine, ketorolac, and morphine, which is administered at the end of the procedure. Intraoperative total knee injections, by contributing to a decrease in postoperative knee pain, may improve early range of motion following TKR.[54,55] The efficacy of periarticular drug infiltration in primary THR has also been documented in the literature.[56,57] Periarticular injection during THR has also demonstrated improved early pain management, reduced need for narcotics, and improved recovery with a shorter length of stay.

IMMEDIATE POSTOPERATIVE PAIN MANAGEMENT

Multimodal anesthesia is also a critical component of postoperative pain management following TJR. Historically, patients were administered significant doses of morphine or narcotic pain medication routinely following TJR. Intravenous patient-controlled analgesia (PCA) was also a common modality for managing pain in the postoperative period.[58] Side effects and complications such as respiratory depression, constipation, and delirium, among others, are frequently associated with the use of intravenous narcotics.[58] In addition, patient participation in postoperative rehabilitation and physical therapy may be limited by the somnolence, nausea, and the physical constraints associated with intravenous PCA, which may promote stiffness, poor mobility, and greater length of stay. To help avoid these potential issues, more modern pain management protocols have focused on oral administration of pain medications and multimodal regimens to minimize narcotics and potential side effects. Multimodal pain management regimens following TJR typically include scheduled doses of acetaminophen up to 4000 mg/d in patients who are able to tolerate this medication safely. In addition, Celebrex 200 to 400 mg/d is also administered for up to 6 weeks postoperatively for its analgesic and antiinflammatory effects. The efficacy of celecoxib was recently demonstrated in a prospective randomized study, which indicated significantly better results 1 year following TKR in patient receiving celecoxib for 6 weeks following surgery.[59] COX-2 inhibitors are chosen because of the lowered potential for antiplatelet effects and lowered risk of bleeding and hematoma formation when compared with nonselective NSAIDs, which are generally contraindicated in the perioperative period. COX-2 inhibitors are used with caution in patients at risk for renal or GI toxicity or where other significant medical contraindications may exist. Gabapentin, a medication with nerve stabilizing properties, is frequently also added in patients with high medication requirements preoperatively and those at risk for neuropathic pain. Initial dosage is 100 to 300 mg up to three times a day; however, the medication may be sedating in some patients.

Oral narcotic medications are also used as an adjunct to these other measures, although there is some evidence that select patients undergoing THR can be successfully treated with only the measures already described.[60,61] The majority of patients undergoing THR and nearly all patients undergoing TKR will receive some form of oral narcotics in the immediate postoperative period. Dilaudid or oxycodone is most commonly used with variable dosage based on patient age, size, and prior tolerance for narcotic pain medication. Patients generally are administered the medication on an as-needed basis every 3 to 6 hours for the first 2 weeks after surgery and then weaning from narcotic medications is begun as pain subsides. Pain medication administration is critical for successful physical therapy following joint replacement surgery, and overaggressive weaning is to be avoided because it can be associated with joint stiffness and withdrawal symptoms. Physical therapy following TKR is particularly critical to the immediate and long-term results, and therefore appropriate pain management including all pharmacologic modalities should be continued until appropriate range of motion has been restored.

SUMMARY

There are many effective treatment measures for OA of the hip or knee, with varying degrees of effectiveness. Nonoperative measures include patient education, physical therapy, activity modification, weight loss, and medications. Pharmacologic strategies include acetaminophen, NSAIDs, injections of cortisone or viscosupplementation, and, less commonly, tramadol or other pain relievers. In patients who may be candidates for TJR, narcotic medications should be avoided to preserve their benefits for the postoperative period.

Over the past 20 years, multimodal pain management has been beneficial to the patient undergoing TJR surgery. Studies have shown this form of pain management decreases postoperative opioid consumption and the related adverse effects. Research is warranted in the areas of postoperative pain scores and patient satisfaction as institutional multimodal protocols continue to evolve.

REFERENCES

1. Iorio R, Robb WJ, Healy WL, et al. Orthopaedic surgeon workforce and volume assessment for total hip and knee replacement in the United States: preparing for an epidemic. J Bone Joint Surg Am 2008;90:1598–605.
2. Kurtz SM, Ong K, Lau E, et al. Projections of primary and revision hip and knee arthroplasty in the United States from 2005 to 2030. J Bone Joint Surg Am 2007;89: 780–5.
3. Ali, M, Pagnano MW, Horlocker T, et al. How I manage pain after total hip arthroplasty. Semin Arthroplasty 2008;231–6.
4. Kehlet H, Dahl JB. The value of multimodal or balanced analgesia in postoperative pain treatment. Anesth Analg 1993;77:1048–56.

5. Zhang W, Moskowitz RW, Nuki G, et al. OARSI recommendations for the management of hip and knee arthritis, part I: critical appraisal of existing treatment guidelines and systematic review of current research evidence. Osteoarthritis Cartilage 2007; 15(9):981–1000.

6. Roddy E, Zhang W, Doherty M, et al. Evidence-based recommendations for the role of exercise in the management of osteoarthritis of the hip or knee–the MOVE consensus. Rheumatology 2005;44:67–73.

7. Ottawa panel evidence-based clinical practice guidelines for therapeutic exercises and manual therapy in the management of osteoarthritis. Phys Therapy 2005;85(9): 907.

8. Hochberg MC, Altman RD, Brandt KD, et al. Guidelines for the medical management of osteoarthritis. Part I. Osteoarthritis of the hip. American College of Rheumatology. Arthritis Rheum 1995;38:1535–40.

9. Garzione JE. Pharmacology and physical therapy intervention for pain management. Gerinotes 2011;18(4):38–40.

10. Perneger TV, Whelton PK, Klag MJ, Risk of kidney failure associated with the use of acetaminophen, ASA and nonsteroidal anti-inflammatory drugs. N Engl J Med 1994; 331:1975–9.

11. Chan AT, Manson JE, Albert CM, et al. Nonsteroidal anti-inflammatory drugs, acetaminophen and the risk for cardiovascular events. Circulation 2006;113:1578–87.

12. Bradley J, Brandt K, Katz B, et al. Comparison of an anti-inflammatory dose of ibuprofen, an analgesic dose of ibuprofen and acetaminophen in the treatment of patients with osteoarthritis of the knee. N Engl J Med 1991;325:87–91.

13. Pincus T, Koch G, Lei H, et al. Patient preference for placebo, acetaminophen or celecoxib efficacy studies (PACES): two randomized, double-blind, placebo controlled, crossover clinical trials in patients with knee or hip osteoarthritis. Ann Rheum Dis 2004;63(8):931–9.

14. Eustice C. Cyclooxygenase: COX-1 and COX-2 explained. What you need to know about Cyclooxygenase. Available at: http://osteoarthritis.about.com/od/osteoarthritismedications/a/cyclooxygenase.htm. Accessed May 11, 2012.

15. Adams ME, Atkinson MH, Lussier AJ, et al. The role of viscosupplementation with hylan G-F 20 in treatment of osteoarthritis of the knee: a Canadian multicenter trial comparing hylan G-F 20 alone, hylan G-F 20 with non-steroidal anti-inflammatory drugs and NSAIDs alone. Osteoarthritis Cartilage 1995;3:213–25.

16. Saleh KJ, Wood KC, Gafni A, et al. Immediate surgery versus waiting list policy in revision total hip arthroplasty. An economic evaluation. J Arthroplasty 1997;12:1–10.

17. Niethard FU, Gold MS, Solomon GS, et al. Efficacy of topical diclofenac diethylamine gel in osteoarthritis of the knee. J Rheumatol 2005;32(12):2384–92.

18. Argoff CE, Gloth FM. Topical non-steroidal anti-inflammatory drugs for management of osteoarthritis in long-term care patients. Ther Clin Risk Manag 2011;7:393–9.

19. Schnitzer TJ. Non-NSAID pharmacologic treatment options for the management of chronic pain. Am J Med 1998;105:45S–52S.

20. Dalacorte RR, Rigo JC, Dalacorte A. Pain management in the elderly at the end of life. N Am J Med Sci 2011;3(8):348–54.

21. Zywiel MG, Stroh DA, Lee SY, et al. Chronic opioid use prior to total knee arthroplasty. J Bone Joint Surg Am 2011;93:1988–93.

22. Harvey WF, Hunter DJ. Pharmacologic intervention for osteoarthritis in older adults. Clin Geriatr Med 2010;26:503–15.

23. Katz WA. Pharmacology and clinical experience with tramadol in osteoarthritis. Drugs 1996;52(Suppl 3):39–47.

24. Parvizi J, Miller AG, Gandhi K. Multimodal pain management after total joint arthroplasty. J Bone Joint Surg Am 2011;93:1075–84.
25. Petrone D, Kamin M, Olson W. Slowing the titration rate of tramadol HCl reduces the incidence of discontinuation due to nausea and/or vomiting: a double blind randomized trial. J Clin Pharm Ther 1999;24:115–23.
26. Ruoff GE. Slowing the initial titration rate of tramadol improves tolerability. Pharmacotherapy 1999;19:88–93.
27. Saxne T, Heinegard D, Wollheim FA et al. Therapeutic effects on cartilage metabolism in arthritis as measured by release of proteoglycan structures into the synovial fluid. Ann Rheum Dis 1986;45:491–7.
28. Armstrong RD, English J, Gibson T, et al. Serum methylprednisolone levels following intra-articular injections of methylprednisolone acetate. Ann Rheum Dis 1981;40:571–4.
29. Dieppe PA, Sathapatayavongs B, Jones HE, et al. Intraarticular steroids in osteoarthritis. Rheumatol Rehabil 1908;19:212–7.
30. Friedman DM, Moore ME. The efficacy of intraarticular steroids in osteoarthritis: a double blind study. J Rheumatol 1980;7:850–6.
31. Valtonen EJ. Clinical comparison of triamcinolone hexacetonide and betamethasone in the treatment of osteoarthritis of the knee joint. Scan J Rheumatol 1981;41(Suppl):3–7.
32. Clemmesen S. Triamcinolone hexacetonide in intraarticular and intramuscular therapy. Acta Rheumatol Scan 1971;17:273–8.
33. Miller JH, White J, Norton TH, et al. The value of intraarticular injection in osteoarthritis of the knee. J Bone Joint Surg Am 1958;40:636–43.
34. Nallamshetty L, Buchowski JM, Nazarian LA, et al. Septic arthritis of the hip following cortisone injection: case report and review of the literature. Clin Imaging. 2003;27(4):225–8.
35. McIntosh AL, Hanssen AD, Wenger DE, et al. Recent intraarticular steroid injection may increase infection rates in primary THA. Clin Orthop Relat Res 2006;451:50–4.
36. Kaspar S, de V de Beer J. Infection in hip arthroplasty after previous injection of steroid. J Bone Joint Surg Br 2005;87:454–7.
37. Balazs EA, Denlinger JL. Viscosupplementation: a new concept in the treatment of osteoarthritis. J Rheumatol 1993;20(Suppl 39):3–9.
38. Bellamy N, Campbell J, Robinson V, et al. Visco-supplementation for treatment of osteoarthritis of the knee. Cochrane Database Syst Rev 2006;2:CD005321.
39. Arrich J, Piribauer F, Mad P, et al. Intra-articular hyaluronic acid for treatment of osteoarthritis of the knee: systematic review and meta-analysis. CMAJ 2005;172:1039–42.
40. Lo GH, LaValley M, McAlindon T, et al. Intra-articular hyaluronic acid in treatment of knee osteoarthritis. A meta-analysis. JAMA 2003;290:3115–21.
41. Altman RD, Moskowitz RW. Intraarticular sodium hyaluronate (Hyalgan) in the treatment of patients with OA of the knee: a randomized clinical trial. J Rheumatol 1998;25:2203–12.
42. Ozturk C, Atamaz F, Hepguler S, et al. The safety and efficacy of intraarticular hyaluronan with/without corticosteroid in knee osteoarthritis: 1-year, single blind, randomized study. Rheumatol Int 2006;26:314–9.
43. Goldberg VM, Coutts RD. Pseudoseptic reaction to hylan viscosupplementation: diagnosis and treatment. Clin Orthop Relat Res 2004;419:130–7.
44. Horlocker T. Pain management in total joint arthroplasty: a historical review. Orthopedics 2010;33:14–9.
45. Dalury DF, Lieberman JR, MacDonald SJ. Current and innovative pain management techniques in total knee arthroplasty. J Bone Joint Surg Am 2011;93:1938–43.

46. Sinatra RS, Torres J, Bustos AM. Pain management after major orthopedic surgery: current strategies and new concepts. J Am Acad Orthop Surg 2002;10:117–29.

47. Dalury DF, Kelley T, Adams MJ. Efficacy of multimodal perioperative analgesia protocol with periarticular drug injection in total knee arthroplasty: a randomized, double blind study. Poster presented at the annual meeting of the American Academy of Orthopedic Surgeons. San Diego, California, February 15–19, 2011.

48. Williams-Russo P, Sharrock NE, Mattis S, et al. Cognitive effects after epidural versus general anesthesia in older adults. A randomized trial. JAMA 1995;27:44–50.

49. Williams-Russo P, Sharrock NE, Haas SB, et al. randomized trial of epidural versus general anesthesia. Outcomes after primary total knee replacement. Clin Orthop Relat Res 1996;331:199–208.

50. Horlocker TT, Cabanela ME, Wedel DJ. Does postoperative epidural analgesia increase the risk of peroneal nerve palsy after total knee arthroplasty? Anesth Analg 1994;79:495–500.

51. Modig J. Spinal or epidural anesthesia with low molecular weight heparin for thromboprophylaxis requires careful postoperative neurological observation. Acta Anaesthesiol Scand 1992;36:603–4.

52. Vandermeulen EP, Van Aken H, Vermylen J. Anticoagulants and spinal-epidural anesthesia. Anesth Analg 1994;79:1165–77.

53. Edwards ND, Wright EM. Continuous low-dose 3-in-1 nerve blockade for postoperative pain relief after total knee replacement. Anesth Analg 1992;75:265–7.

54. Joo JH, Park JW, Kim JS, et al. Is intra-articular multimodal drug injection effective in pain management after total knee arthroplasty? J Arthroplasty 2011;26:1095–9.

55. Fajardo M, Collins J, Landa J, et al. Effect of a perioperative intra-articular injection on pain control and early range of motion following bilateral TKA. Orthopedics 2011;34: 354–8.

56. Banerjee P, McLean C. The efficacy of multimodal high volume wound infiltration in primary hip replacement. Orthopedics 2011;34:522–9.

57. Busch CA, Whitehouse MR, Shore BJ, et al. The efficacy of periarticular multimodal drug infiltration in total hip arthroplasty. Clin Orthop Relat Res 2010;468:2152–9.

58. Singelyn FJ, Deyaert M, Joris D, et al. Effects of intravenous patient-controlled analgesia with morphine, continuous epidural analgesia, and continuous three-in-one block on postoperative pain and knee rehabilitation after unilateral total knee arthroplasty. Anaesth Analg 1998;87:88–92.

59. Schroer WC, Diesfeld PJ, LeMarr AR, et al. Benefits of prolonged postoperative cyclooxygenase-2 inhibitor administration on total knee arthroplasty recovery. J Arthroplasty 2011;26(Suppl 1):2–7.

60. Maheshwari AV, Boutary M, Yun AG, et al. Multimodal analgesia without routine parental narcotics for total hip arthroplasty. Clin Orthop Relat Res 2006;453:231–8.

61. Dorr LD, Maheshwari AV, Aditya V, et al. Early pain relief and function after posterior minimally invasive and conventional total hip arthroplasty: a prospective, randomized, blinded study. J Bone Joint Surg Am 2007;89:1153–60.

Perioperative Complications Following Total Joint Replacement

Carl T. Talmo, MD*, Mehran Aghazadeh, MD, James V. Bono, MD

KEYWORDS

- Total knee arthroplasty • Total hip arthroplasty • Complications

KEY POINTS

- Total joint replacement (TJR) of the hip and knee is an extremely effective procedure resulting in decreased pain and improved function in patients who have osteoarthritis. Utilization of TJR is increasing at a significant rate, and increased awareness of potential complications following TJR is of paramount importance to all practitioners.
- The geriatric patient may be more susceptible to some perioperative complications following TJR; therefore, careful preoperative planning, close perioperative monitoring, and the institution of appropriate preventative measures will help to minimize complications and dampen their impact on elderly patients when they do occur.
- Important complications to consider in the elderly patient following TJR include infection, thromboembolism, fracture, hip dislocation, and delirium, as well as cardiovascular complications.

INTRODUCTION

Total joint replacement (TJR) has become an extremely effective and successful treatment for osteoarthritis (OA) of the hip and knee. The procedures are among the most successful procedures available in medicine as quantified by a number of measures.[1-8] There is also substantial evidence that elderly patients undergoing TJR receive these benefits along with an associated decrease in health care costs compared with usual care.[9] Advances in technology, surgical technique, and perioperative care over the past few decades have made total hip replacement (THR) and total knee arthroplasty (TKA) more suitable for a wider age group of patients, including the very elderly.[3-5]

The association between OA and aging is well known.[9-11] OA of the hip and knee typically causes significant and progressive pain along with deterioration in function, ambulation, and mobility and is a leading cause of physical disability in the elderly population.[9] OA of the hip and knee is the most common musculoskeletal disorder in

Disclosures: The authors did not receive any outside funding or grants in support of their research for or preparation of this work.
New England Baptist Hospital, Tufts University, 125 Parker Hill Avenue, Boston, MA 02120, USA
* Corresponding author.

this age group, accounting for up to 60% of musculoskeletal complaints in the population over age 64 in some reports.[9]

Seniors are the fastest growing population worldwide. Statistics from the US Census Bureau confirm the number of Americans over age 65 has increased by a factor of 12, from 3.1 million in 1900 to 38.9 million in 2008.[12] The fastest growing segment of the elderly population is those 85 years of age or over. This small segment of the population is projected to reach 19 million worldwide by 2050.[12] This rapid increase in the elderly population is expected to have a significant impact on the utilization and economic burden of health care in the United States. This increase is particularly apparent in the cost associated with the treatment of musculoskeletal disease.

Because of these and other factors, primary THR and total knee replacement (TKR) procedures have increased steadily between 1990 and 2002, and the rate is projected to increase substantially over the next two decades.[13,14] Within the United States it is expected that the demand for total hip arthroplasty will increase 174% by the year 2030, and total knee arthroplasty could be as high as 3.48 million procedures.[14] The logistic and economic impact of these projections is substantial and will likely require a widespread understanding of the procedures and their perioperative care among all health care providers.

Patients with significant pain and functional disability due to OA of the hip and knee are candidates for referral for TJR. First line treatment of OA includes acetaminophen or nonsteroidal antiinflammatory medications (NSAIDs) and weight loss, as well as consideration for use of a cane.[10] Physical therapy for quadriceps strengthening and water exercises may be beneficial in the treatment of knee OA.[9,10] Corticosteroid injection may be valuable for short-term relief of a painfully swollen arthritic knee, whereas viscosupplementation therapies remain controversial.[15] There is little role for the use of cortisone injection in the hip.[16] Use of NSAIDs is associated with significant morbidity and toxicity in the elderly population, most notably a high rate of bleeding and peptic ulcer disease, and therefore must be monitored closely.[15] Patients at risk for side effects associated with the use of oral medications such as NSAIDs are candidates for earlier referral and consideration for TJR.[10] The risks and potential complications of these nonoperative treatments may be significant and should be taken into account in comparison with the effectiveness and relatively low rate of complications associated with TJR.

THR is one of the most successful interventions in medicine.[8,17,18] The procedure is essentially unrivaled in surgery in terms of its success rates and patient satisfaction.[8] Numerous studies have demonstrated improved pain, function, and quality of life following THR for several decades.[1–8,19] Using functional scoring systems and validated outcome measurements such as the short form-36 and the Western Ontario and McMaster University Osteoarthritis Index, a number of researchers have consistently shown significant improvement in health-related quality of life following THR.[2,6] The degree of improvement in these scores for both hip and knee arthroplasty has also been shown to be significant and dramatic in effect when compared with traditional nonoperative or conservative measures.[5] Whereas comorbid illnesses can influence the results, this improvement has been noted across all age groups, and age has not been found to be an obstacle to successful surgery and outcomes.[2] A number of studies have also demonstrated excellent results in the elderly population, with low risks and complication rates even in comparison with more youthful populations.[4,20–22]

TKA is one of the most highly successful and commonly performed orthopedic procedures in the United States. For the past 40 years, TKA has proved to be an efficacious treatment for persons with OA in relieving pain and restoring function.[2,3,7] There is extensive literature to support the efficacy of TKR in the elderly.[3,5,9,11,20,23–25] Careful consideration should be paid to preoperative systemic disease, hearing or vision deficits, psychological status, living arrangements, and patient expectations. With careful consideration and preoperative planning, treating the very elderly patient is typically safe and successful, and therefore advanced age should not be a limiting factor for knee replacement surgery.[20,23–25] A number of studies have reviewed the results of TKR in a group of patients over age 75 to 80 years and noted excellent patient satisfaction, pain relief, stability, and range of motion, comparable with a group of younger patients undergoing the procedure.[3,19,25] Significant improvements in health outcome have been documented in these patients including improved pain, emotional reaction, sleep, and physical mobility as early as 3 to 12 months after the operation.[3,26] In comparison with younger patients, TKR provides equivalent pain relief, functional improvement, strength, stability, and range of motion. The procedure is also equally cost-effective in both younger and older patient groups.[26] In a retrospective study, Hosick and colleagues[27] found a higher rate of early postoperative medical complications in patients over 80 years undergoing TKR, but still significant pain relief and functional improvement following recovery.

COMPLICATIONS AND SPECIAL CONSIDERATIONS FOLLOWING TJR IN THE ELDERLY

TJRs are safe procedures with a relatively low rate of complications. Although there is some evidence that elderly patients may be at higher risk for medical and surgical complications following surgery, the evidence is conflicting. Smaller scale retrospective studies have indicated higher rates of mortality and complication rates in the elderly.[19,21,27,28] A larger scale study of Medicare claims data indicated that older age was a risk factor for an adverse outcome within 90 days following THR including death, dislocation, and infection.[18] Some reports indicate a higher rate of mortality, cardiopulmonary complications, hip dislocation, urinary tract infection (UTI), and other perioperative infectious complications following surgery in the elderly.[18,21,29] Phillips and colleagues[30] reviewed perioperative complications in patients over 80 undergoing THR including death, postoperative myocardial infarction (MI), thromboembolism, UTI, and postoperative confusion and found that complications and postoperative morbidity correlated significantly with the American Society of Anesthesiologists (ASA) score. Patients with an ASA rating of III or higher had a 15% risk of perioperative complication, significantly greater than those with an ASA class I or II.[30]

More recent studies have demonstrated lower rates of postoperative complications across the board in TJR, most likely due to increased awareness and medical screening that has correlated with the increased volume of elective joint replacement occurring throughout the world.[18] In a review of over 10,000 patients undergoing elective TJR, the overall rate of adverse events within 30 days of surgery was 2.2% including MI (0.4%), pulmonary embolism (PE) (0.7%), deep vein thrombosis (DVT) (1.5%), and death (0.5%), and the frequency of these events did increase with age, particularly for patients aged 70 years or older.[30] Other case-control and comparative studies have found complication rates and mortality more comparable with other age groups undergoing TJR.[22,26] Certainly complication rates in both groups are low, but based on these results, careful perioperative monitoring of elderly patients is warranted to aid in the prevention of complications.

Additional risk factors may place certain patients at higher risk for complications following TJR. Increased risk for infection among diabetic patients is well-established; more recent research has also identified that diabetic patients are at increased risk for other complications as well.[31,32] Diabetic patients are at increased risk for PE, stroke, UTI, ileus, postoperative hemorrhage, and death. Improving perioperative glycemic

---

Box 1
Complications following TJR

1. Thromboembolism
2. Infection
3. Periprosthetic fracture
4. MI/congestive heart failure
5. Neurovascular injury
6. Periprosthetic loosening
7. Instability/dislocation
8. Stiffness

---

control can reduce the incidence of these complications in the diabetic population, and preoperative assessment of glycemic control in diabetic patients in recommended.[31]

Patients with rheumatoid arthritis are at increased risk for postoperative joint infection following prosthetic replacement. Because of osteopenia associated with this disease, these patients are also at increased risk for periprosthetic fracture. Patients with chronic renal insufficiency may be at higher risk of infection or hemorrhage, as well as prosthetic loosening leading to revision surgery.[32,33]

Elderly patients undergoing THR for the treatment of hip fracture are at increased risk for postoperative complications when compared with patients undergoing THR on an elective basis. These patients are at increased risk for medical complications including cardiac events, thromboembolism, infection, and death, as well as an increased risk of hip dislocation.[30,34]

There is also evidence that patients undergoing TJR by surgeons who perform a low volume of the procedures or at lower volume institutions are at increased risk for postoperative complications, even including thromboembolism and death.[35,36] Although there may be inherent differences in the populations that choose to undergo surgery in a higher volume versus a lower volume center resulting in a possible selection bias in some of these studies, there are a number of studies that indicate higher complication rates among lower volume surgeons and institutions.[37,38]

Certain potential complications in the elderly deserve special consideration so that appropriate prevention strategies may be used without introducing additional morbidity (**Box 1**). These are reviewed in further detail.

PERIPROSTHETIC JOINT INFECTION

Infection rates vary from about .2% to 2.5% following elective TJR.[39–45] The risk of infection is slightly higher in TKR when compared with THR.[43] Risk factors for infection include age, diabetes mellitus, rheumatoid arthritis, a history of prior surgery on the joint, chronic infection elsewhere in the body, chronic kidney or liver disease, malnutrition, steroid use, smoking, and early wound complications or hematoma.[38–45] Other risk factors may include a higher ASA score, morbid obesity, allogenic blood transfusion, postoperative atrial fibrillation, MI, and prolonged hospitalization.[43]

There is increasing evidence that prolonged wound bleeding and drainage, hematoma formation at the surgical site, and reoperation for evacuation of hematoma place a patient at increased risk for deep infection.[44] For this reason, wound care and monitoring by the physician, nursing staff, and therapists are imperative following TJR, and careful consideration must be given to postoperative anticoagulation along with this care and monitoring.

Preoperative screening is an integral part of infection prevention in TJR. There is increasing evidence that screening patients' nares for the presence of staphylococcus aureus and methicillin-resistant *Staphylococcus aureus* (MRSA) aids in lowering infection rate following TJR. At the authors' institution a strict screening protocol is followed for all patients undergoing TJR.[46] Patients receive a nasal swab at their prescreening visit prior to surgery, and patients identified as carriers of these organisms are treated with intranasal Bactroban prior to the surgery. Patients identified as carriers of MRSA are also treated with vancomycin for perioperative antibiotic prophylaxis, and patients who are unable to clear MRSA colonization from their nares prior to surgery are also treated with gown and glove precautions in a private room during their hospitalization. This protocol has reduced the rate of postoperative infection by greater than 50% from .45% to .19%, including a reduction in MRSA infection.[46]

Routine use of intravenous antibiotics covering gram-positive bacteria preoperatively and for the first 24 hours postoperatively has been shown to aid in the prevention of infection and in reducing postoperative infection rates; however, continuing antibiotics beyond 24 hours has not been shown to be beneficial.[39] The most common pathogenic bacteria in periprosthetic infections are skin flora including staph epidermidis, now the most common, and S aureus. First-generation cephalosporins are the most commonly used prophylactic antibiotics, with vancomycin as an alternative in patients with a history of cephalosporin allergy or a history of MRSA colonization.[41]

Periprosthetic joint infections may be superficial or deep; however, to avoid the devastating complication of chronic deep infection, all infections should be considered deep until proven otherwise.[41] Routine administration of oral antibiotics for reddened wounds, a common finding after even uncomplicated joint replacement surgeries, is strongly discouraged in lieu of further careful assessment for infection and holding any antibiotics until actual causative bacteria are identified.[41,44]

The signs and symptoms of periprosthetic infection include increased pain, stiffness, prolonged or excessive wound drainage, or dehiscence, and rarely fever or constitutional symptoms as well. In the elderly or immunocompromised patient the presentation may be subtle until the infection becomes severe and fulminant.[41] Many patients presenting with infection have only pain as the sole presenting symptom. Evaluation for the presence of infection begins with laboratory testing for C-reactive protein (CRP) and erythrocyte sedimentation rate (ESR).[47,48] In combination, these tests have a very high sensitivity for the diagnosis of periprosthetic joint infection. In the setting of an elevated CRP and/or ESR, joint aspiration testing should be considered. All aspirations should be sent for Gram stain and culture of the synovial fluid, which may demonstrate bacterial growth; however, false-negative results are common, and studies have demonstrated a sensitivity of only 50% to 86% for culture testing of joint aspirations.[48] Antibiotic administration can contaminate these results, and therefore antibiotics should always be held until appropriate joint fluid analysis can be performed when a periprosthetic joint infection is suspected. Joint fluid analysis for cell count and differential has a much higher sensitivity and specificity for periprosthetic joint infection, and it is imperative that all joint aspirates include testing for cell count and differential whenever possible. Joint aspirates containing greater than 1100 nucleated cells/10 cm^3 and less than 64% neutrophils on the differential are essentially considered diagnostic for infection in a TJR with an accuracy of approximately 98.6%. Conversely, aspirates containing cell counts and differentials lower than these numbers can be considered free of infection.[49] These numbers are much lower than those considered suspicious for infection in native joints.

The treatment of infections follows a fairly complex algorithm, which typically involves surgical intervention for successful eradication.[41,47] Treatment of infections considered superficial or acute includes surgical debridement with retention of the prosthesis and culture-specific intravenous antibiotics. This procedure typically involves removal and exchange of only the modular portions of the prosthesis such as the polyethylene liner and therefore is colloquially referred to as "liner exchange." The results of these procedures are quite variable based on the chronicity of infection, the bacterial strain, and a number of other variables, with success rates as low as 30% to 50%; however, the procedure has a low early morbidity and therefore is widely accepted as a treatment strategy for many patients.[47]

Infections considered chronic and deep are treated with complete surgical revision, sometimes in a single procedure but much more commonly in two stages followed by intravenous culture-specific antibiotics[41,47] **(Fig. 1)**. Two-stage revision surgery has the highest success rate for eradication of infection, with success rates commonly

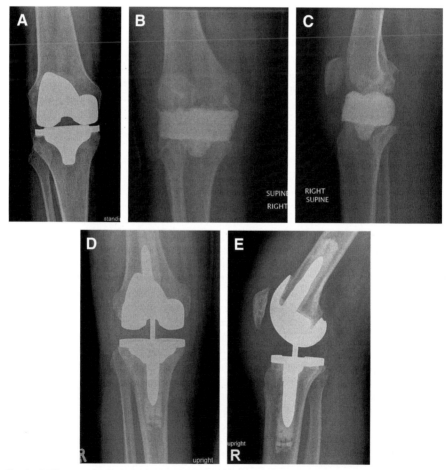

Fig. 1. A 78-year-old man presents with a late chronic infection 18 months following TKR (A). The patient undergoes two-stage revision surgery with resection of the TKR and placement and antibiotic-impregnated cement spacer (B, C). Following a 6-week course of culture-specific intravenous antibiotics followed by repeat testing to be sure that infection was eradicated, the second-stage reimplantation procedure is performed (D, E).

reported between 93% and 95%; however, the procedure has a significant period of convalescence and greater blood loss and may have a greater overall morbidity.[47] The exact definition of what constitutes an acute versus chronic infection is somewhat controversial. Infections occurring within a month or so of surgery are generally considered early acute infections. In addition, infections presenting in a fulminant fashion in a previously well-functioning TJR, presumably seeded from an episode of bacteremia, are also considered acute when there have been symptoms for less than 4 weeks, and these types of infections may be termed *acute metastatic infection* or *acute bacteremic infections*. Infections presenting with roughly more than 4 weeks of symptoms are generally considered chronic.[47]

In the elderly patient with a poor life expectancy, chronic oral suppressive antibiotics, alone or in combination with a more simple surgical debridement procedure (such as liner exchange), may be an appropriate treatment for sensitive low-virulence organisms, particularly when the risks associated with revision surgery or removal of the prosthesis are considerable.[41,47]

THROMBOEMBOLIC DISEASE AND PREVENTION

The incidence of DVT following TJR with prophylaxis is extremely low.[50] Following elective TJR with modern prophylaxis regimens, the rate of symptomatic DVT varies around 1% to 2%, with a higher rate of DVT seen after TKR.[50] The rate of symptomatic PE with these regimens ranges from 0% to .5% and is slightly higher following THR.[50] Prophylaxis against thromboembolism is therefore universally recommended. Agents commonly used in some combination include mechanical measures (compression stockings; lower leg or foot pneumatic compression boots), injectable low-molecular-weight heparins (LMWH), injectable synthetic pentasaccharides or factor Xa inhibitors, variable dose warfarin, or fixed low-dose warfarin and aspirin.[50–52] Most prophylaxis regimens are continued for only 10 days to 6 weeks postoperatively.[50] When choosing a regimen for prophylaxis, the surgeon must balance the risk of thromboembolism against the risk of bleeding and hematoma formation and the potential for infection at the surgical site.[51] Risk factors for thromboembolic complications include a history of prior DVT or PE, advanced age, congestive heart failure, MI, stroke, obesity, and hypercoagulable states.[50,51] Easily overlooked when choosing a form of prophylaxis are preexisting risk factors for bleeding or hemorrhage including history of bleeding disorder, gastrointestinal (GI) bleeding, hemorrhagic stroke, or other risks.[51] Elderly patients may be at higher risk for GI complications or hemorrhagic stroke as well as having a higher potential for falls in the postoperative period, placing them at risk for soft tissue hematomas and intracranial or subdural bleeding.

The American Academy of Orthopedic Surgeons (AAOS), in coordination with other public health organizations, has made practice guidelines based on a thorough review of the existing literature.[51] These recommendations support preoperative risk assessment for PE as well as bleeding and selection of a thromboprophylactic regimen that aims for a balance between safety and efficacy and takes into account a patient's risk of bleeding as well as risk for thromboembolism. Based on this balance, the AAOS has found sufficient evidence to support the following chemotherapeutic regimens following TKR and THR: aspirin, LMWH, synthetic pentasaccharides, and variable-dose warfarin with a goal international normalized ratio at or below 2.0.[51] For patients at higher risk of PE and a standard risk of major bleeding, aspirin was not recommended, whereas for patients at a standard risk for PE and increased risk of major bleeding, LMWH and synthetic pentasaccharides were not recommended because these have been shown to result in a increased risk of bleeding, hematoma, and wound drainage, which may influence the development of a deep joint infection.[44,51] At the authors' own institution, they have had success with a fixed low-dose regimen of warfarin (1 mg) for 6 weeks following elective THR in patients at standard risk for postoperative thromboembolism, obviating the need for blood draws, with results comparable with all other agents in terms of safety and efficacy.[52]

POSTOPERATIVE DELIRIUM

Postoperative delirium is a common and serious problem in hospitalized elderly patients following elective TJR.[53,54] Patients experiencing postoperative confusion and delirium can be disruptive and distressing to other patients and the health care team but more importantly to themselves, frequently incurring self-inflicted injury or being susceptible to falls. Patients who have experienced delirium may have little or no recollection of the early postoperative period, and this loss of control is frequently disconcerting.[53] Delirium may occur in up to 44% of hospitalized elderly patients after major surgery[54] and in approximately 28% of elderly patients undergoing THR.[55]

The consequences of postoperative delirium including prolonged hospitalization, hip dislocation, immobility with associated skin compromise, infection and thromboembolic risk, falls and injuries, and the potential for impaired rehabilitation and recovery are significant and may be costly to hospitals and the health care system.[53–56] Costs associated with the treatment of postoperative delirium have been estimated at 2.5 times the costs of caring for other patients.[57] Risk factors for postoperative delirium include age, preexisting cognitive impairment or dementia, a history of delirium, and a history of alcohol dependence.[53] A number of preventative strategies have been used including use of regional anesthesia, limiting use of postoperative narcotics, rapid mobilization and return to familiar environments, and antipsychotic medications.[55,56] Medications used in preventing and treating postoperative delirium have included haloperidol, risperidone, donepezil, and olanzapine.[53–55]

In the authors' institution, appropriate at-risk patients undergoing TJR are treated prophylactically with olanzapine pre- and postoperatively with excellent results.[56] A prospective randomized double-blind placebo controlled trial has demonstrated a significant reduction in postoperative delirium in these patients with only 14% of patients in the olanzapine group versus 40% of patients in the placebo group experiencing postoperative delirium. Advanced age, higher ASA class, abnormal albumin levels, and knee replacement surgery were identified as independent risk factors for postoperative delirium.[56]

PERIPROSTHETIC FRACTURE

Fractures occurring around TJRs are a relatively common complication of TJR and can be a major source of morbidity in the elderly. Fractures may occur intraoperatively, in the early postoperative period, or late following TJR.[58] Each of these scenarios is distinctly different, and each requires a different treatment and has potentially different prognosis.

Intraoperative fractures are common in THR with an incidence of between .5% and 10%.[59–62] Rates of intraoperative fracture vary depending on patient factors, the operative setting, surgical technique, and the type of implants used.[63] Certain disease processes may predispose to periprosthetic fracture including rheumatoid arthritis, hip dysplasia, Paget disease, and osteoporosis. Gender has been controversial in past reports, with some studies demonstrating an increased risk of intraoperative fracture in women. A history of anemia or thalassemia has also been suggested to increase the risk of intraoperative fracture.[58] Periprosthetic fracture is significantly more common during or following revision TJR.[58,63–65] The increasing use of cementless implants has been accompanied by an increased rate of fracture, because these implants rely on a very tight fit with cortical bone to achieve a lasting degree of fixation.[58,64] When sizing and inserting these components, there can be a fine line between what constitutes an appropriate fit and one that results in the initiation of a fracture. In a series of primary THRs from the Mayo clinic, intraoperative fracture was .3% with cemented implants and 5.4% using cementless, and the rate of fracture was also much higher in revision surgery (20.9%).[64]

Intraoperative fractures are typically noted by the surgeon and treated appropriately during the procedure, resulting in little or no change in the ultimate prognosis. Intraoperative femoral fracture during THR is the most common and is typically treated by the application of cerclage wires and protected weightbearing postoperatively with mainly good results.[58–60]

Fractures occurring in the early postoperative period (1–3 months) can occur with a subtle injury or fall and frequently require reoperation or revision surgery (**Fig. 2**). During this period the bone is healing to the metal implant and the bond is incomplete, making the bone somewhat more susceptible to fracture when the metal stem is subjected to either an abnormal degree of torsional or axial force, literally splitting the bone. If these fractures are nondisplaced and the implant remains stable within the bone, the patient may be treated nonoperatively with a period of careful protected weightbearing until the fracture is healed.[66] Fractures that are displaced are typically treated with surgical fixation and frequently revision of the components if they are loose. When these fractures do occur, there is a significant risk that revision surgery, ultimately for implant loosening, will be required.[61]

Late periprosthetic fractures (occurring more than 3 months postoperatively) are a common cause of revision surgery in the elderly. The majority of these patients will have poor results when treated with nonoperative measures such as traction, bed rest, casting, or protected weightbearing alone.[61] These fractures are typically treated with surgical fixation or revision or a combination of the procedures. Elderly patients who sustain these injuries are at significant risk for complications associated with trauma and immobility, and there is evidence that expedient surgical treatment of these patients improves survival and lessens morbidity.[67]

DISLOCATION FOLLOWING THR

Perhaps the most feared complication following THR, dislocation has historically been one of the more common complications after TJR. Incidence of dislocation following THR has varied widely in past reports, ranging from .3% to 10% of patients. A large-scale study of the Medicare population demonstrated a 3.9% incidence of dislocation in the first 6 months following THR.[34] Other investigators have reported a lifetime risk of dislocation of 4.8% following THR, with the majority of dislocations occurring many years after the surgery.[68] It is no surprise that a number of patient risk factors and surgical factors dramatically impact a patient's risk for postoperative dislocation. In general, it is widely believed that a number of refinements in the surgical technique and improvements in the technology have resulted in decreased rates of dislocation over the last several years.[69]

Positioning of the implants during the surgery, particularly the acetabular component, is a critical factor in success of the procedure and in avoiding postoperative dislocation.[68–70] The risk of dislocation is also influenced by the surgical approach, with historically higher rates of dislocation for posterior approaches. Surgical approach has become more controversial in recent years as a number of studies have

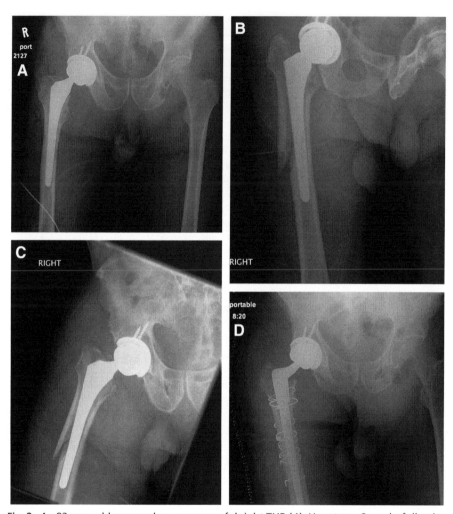

Fig. 2. An 82-year-old man undergoes successful right THR (*A*). He returns 3 weeks following the procedure complaining of pain and difficulty walking after a fall in his rehabilitation hospital during an episode of transient delirium, and radiographs demonstrate a displaced periprosthetic femoral fracture (*B, C*). The patient requires revision to a longer prosthesis with cerclage wiring of the femur (*D*).

demonstrated equivalent or even lower dislocation rates with posterior approaches using strategies to repair or preserve posterior soft tissues.[69] Dislocation is considerably more common following revision surgery, with rates of dislocation approaching 28% in some series.[69,71] Other surgical factors that seem to play a role in the risk of dislocation include the type of prosthesis and the size of the prosthetic femoral head, with larger heads having a lower rate of dislocation.[69]

Preoperative diagnosis also influences the rate of postoperative dislocation because patients with a history of rheumatoid or inflammatory arthritis, posttraumatic arthritis, congenital hip dysplasia, avascular necrosis, or fracture of the hip/proximal femur are at increased risk for dislocation.[68,70] Women and patients over the age of

70 years are also at higher risk.[68] Other risk factors include an altered mental state such as delirium or alcohol use and significant neurologic impairment such as Parkinson disease or spinal cord injury.[69,71]

Most episodes of dislocation are managed nonoperatively with closed reduction procedures either under sedation or general anesthesia. Following closed reduction, certain precautions or restrictions on movement may be instituted in patients capable of following instructions. A period of bracing may also be warranted to prevent early recurrence.[69] Irreducible dislocations require surgical intervention and frequently revision surgery. After three episodes of dislocation, the risk of continued episode of dislocation becomes much more likely, and elective revision surgery is typically advised.[68,69,72] The type of revision surgery performed varies depending on the root cause of dislocation and may range from simple exchange of modular implants to use of a captured liner to revision of the implants to in very severe cases removal of all implants and chronic resection of the hip joint. Success rates of revision surgery for dislocation are quite variable with a significantly better prognosis when a technical reason for dislocation can be identified and improved on.[72]

CARDIOVASCULAR COMPLICATIONS

Despite the fact that TJR is considered major surgery, cardiovascular complications following TJR are relatively rare, and the procedures are considered safe in the vast majority of elderly patients. Estimated incidence of in-hospital cardiovascular complications following TJR are quite low, including arrhythmia 0.6%, acute MI 0.2%, stroke 0.2%, congestive heart failure 0.6%, and death 0.06% to 0.16%.[73–75]

Preoperative screening and risk stratification are warranted in all patients undergoing TJR. All patients over age 50 undergoing elective TJR are screened preoperatively with history, physical examination, complete blood counts, and electrocardiogram. Additional testing may be warranted based on symptoms. Factors associated with a higher risk of cardiac complications include age, a history of arrhythmia, a history of coronary artery disease, MI, congestive heart failure, or valvular heart disease. Other risk factors include revision surgery and bilateral surgery under a single anesthetic.[76] Preoperative cardiology consultation is warranted in patients with a history of these cardiac conditions, as well as in elderly patients whose activity levels are very compromised, such that an assessment of activity-related signs of cardiac disease cannot be determined.

Stroke following TJR is a rare yet devastating complication. In one large series, 25% of patients experiencing stroke after TJR died within 1 year of the procedure. Risk factors for stroke following TJR included noncoronary heart disease, urgent (vs elective) surgery, general (vs regional) anesthesia, and intraoperative arrhythmia or alteration in heart rate.[75]

NEUROVASCULAR INJURY

Vascular injury following modern TJR is exceedingly rare, with an incidence of approximately 0.1% to 2% of all TJR.[77] Patients with a history of peripheral vascular disease appear to be at higher risk for vascular injury in the perioperative period. Patients with absent or severely diminished peripheral pulses and claudication symptoms may require preoperative assessment by a vascular surgeon in the event that vascular bypass or stenting procedures are required prior to TJR.[77,78] When significant vascular disease is suspected in a patient considering TJR, evaluation with an arterial duplex study may assist in screening or staging of occult vascular disease.

Careful monitoring and documentation of pulses are required in the vasculopathic patient perioperatively. Typically tourniquets are avoided in knee replacement surgery in these patients, which may result in a higher intraoperative blood loss but also assists in minimizing trauma to vessels with preexisting disease. When serious vascular injury does occur, the consequences can be devastating, resulting in the need for urgent bypass surgery and a risk of amputation.

Nerve injury is also very rare following TJR, with a reported incidence ranging from 0.17% to 3.7% following THR and 0.3% to 4% following TKR.[79–81] Risk factors for nerve palsy following total hip replacement include a history of developmental dysplasia of the hip, a diagnosis of posttraumatic OA, revision surgery, and significant lengthening of the limb during surgery.[79,80] Patients with rheumatoid arthritis or a history of peripheral neuropathy or spinal stenosis may also be at increased risk.[80] Risk factors for nerve palsy following TKR include severe preoperative valgus deformity and flexion contracture, rheumatoid arthritis, prolonged use of a tourniquet, epidural anesthesia, and a history of neuropathy including nerve root compression due to spinal stenosis.[80] Other factors that may cause or contribute to the development of a perioperative nerve injury include external nerve compression such as a tight bandage, the development of a hematoma, and intraoperative nerve trauma or laceration.[80–82]

Most nerve palsies occurring in the perioperative period are transient neurapraxias that will improve or resolve over time.[80] Most commonly, patients exhibit dysfunction in the peroneal branches of the sciatic nerve because this nerve seems the most susceptible to injury, and a postoperative foot drop is encountered.[80] The vast majority of nerve palsies occurring following total knee replacement have an excellent prognosis for complete or near complete recovery.[81] After THR, the prognosis may not be as good, with significant residual nerve deficit reported in 64% to 81% of patients.[79]

The prevention and management of nerve problems following TJR begins preoperatively with a careful preoperative neurologic examination and appropriate documentation. Even remote nerve palsies that have occurred in the past have been known to recur after surgery, and sometimes subtle neuropathic conditions can be exacerbated by surgery. High-risk patients require careful positioning to avoid external compression, and tourniquet use may be limited in some cases. Regional anesthesia such as spinal or epidural may also be avoided in these cases. Clinical neurologic examination is performed in all patients postoperatively, and in patients with signs of new nerve dysfunction, the limb is carefully positioned to reduce compression and relieve tension on the abnormal nerve. This positioning is most commonly accomplished by slight flexion of the knee when there is alteration in sciatic or peroneal nerve function. Bandages are also loosened to minimize compression. Patients are also evaluated for hematoma by physical examination, with serial blood tests or, less commonly, with imaging studies. Serial examinations are also necessary in the postoperative period to monitor for improvement or signs of progressive worsening. Most nerve palsies resolve with conservative treatment postoperatively, and signs of improvement may be noted within minutes after repositioning whereas others may take months to improve. Further surgical interventions are rarely ever necessary. If a significant hematoma is identified, surgical decompression may be warranted. Other interventions such as electromyogram testing or surgical exploration and the timing of these interventions are somewhat controversial.[80–82]

PERIPROSTHETIC LOOSENING

Loosening of the prosthetic components is typically a late complication and rarely ever occurs within the first year after TJR. A detailed discussion of loosening is beyond the scope of this article. Patients with painful TJRs or patients who fail to make appropriate progress following TJR should be evaluated with radiographs or serial imaging studies to determine if precocious loosening is occurring. These patients should also be carefully evaluated for infection and occult fractures, because these are the most common causes of early or unexpected loosening.

SUMMARY

Total joint arthroplasty is a safe and highly effective treatment for moderate to severe osteoarthritic symptoms and other causes of joint derangement in the elderly population. Significant improvements in pain, function, and quality of life are nearly universal, with a low rate of complications and adverse outcomes. Because of its success and cost-effectiveness, the rate of utilization of TJR is increasing, and all health care providers must be familiar with the potential complications and perioperative management of these patients. Elderly patients may be at a higher risk for postoperative medical complications; however, the majority of these complications are minor and many are avoidable with appropriate preoperative screening and careful postoperative management. As with all patients undergoing TJR, patients should be prophylactically treated for infection and thromboembolism and carefully followed for the development of these potential complications as well as fracture, hip dislocation, and neurovascular dysfunction. Postoperative delirium may be minimized and prophylactically treated in appropriate elderly patients to maximize recovery and promote safety.

REFERENCES

1. Laupacis A, Bourne R, Rorabeck C, et al. The effect of elective total hip replacement on health-related quality of life. J Bone Joint Surg Am 1993;75(11):1619.
2. Ethgen O, Bruyere O, Richy F, et al. Health-related quality of life in total hip and total knee arthroplasty. A qualitative and systematic review of the literature. J Bone Joint Surg Am 2004;86(5):963–74.
3. Birdsall PD, Hayes JH, Cleary R, et al. Health outcome after total knee replacement in the very elderly. J Bone Joint Surg Br 1999;81:660–2.
4. Levy RN, Levy CM, Snyder J, et al. Outcome and long-term results following total hip replacement in elderly patients. Clin Orthop 1995;316:25–30.
5. Hamel MB, Toth M, Legedza A, et al. Joint replacement surgery in elderly patients with severe osteoarthritis of the hip or knee. Arch Int Med 2008;168:1430–40.
6. Hozack J, Rothman RH, Albert TJ, et al. Relationship of total hip arthroplasty outcomes to other orthopedic procedures. Clin Orthop 1997;344:81–7.
7. Ritter MA, Albohm MJ, Keating EM, et al. Comparative outcomes of total joint arthroplasty. J Arthroplasty 1995;10:737–41.
8. Learmonth ID, Young C, Rorabeck C. The operation of the century: total hip replacement. The Lancet 2007;370(9597)1508–19.
9. Lohmander S. Osteoarthritis: a major cause of disability in the elderly. In: Buckwalter JA, Goldwater VM, Woo SL-Y, editors. Musculoskeletal soft-tissue aging: impact on mobility. Rosemont (IL): American Academy of Orthopaedic Surgeons; 1993. p. 99–115.

10. Hochberg MC, Altman RD, Brandt KD, et al. Guidelines for the medical management of osteoarthritis. Part I. Osteoarthritis of the hip. American College of Rheumatology. Arthritis Rheum 1995;38:1535–40.

11. Goldberg VM, Buckwalter JA, Hayes WC, et al. Orthopaedic challenges in an aging population. Instr Course Lect 1997;46:417–22.

12. United States Census Bureau. Population profile, the elderly population. Available at: http://www.census.gov/population/www/pop-profile/elderpop.html. Accessed November 29, 2011.

13. Kurtz SM, Ong KL, Schmier J, et al. Future clinical and economic impact of revision total hip and knee arthroplasty. J Bone Joint Surg Am 2007;89:144–51.

14. Kurtz SM, Ong K, Lau E, et al. Projections of primary and revision hip and knee arthroplasty in the United States from 2005 to 2030. J Bone Joint Surg Am 2007;89: 780–5.

15. Adams ME, Atkinson MH, Lussier AJ, et al. The role of viscosupplementation with hylan G-F 20 in treatment of osteoarthritis of the knee: a Canadian multicenter trial comparing hylan G-F 20 alone, hylan G-F 20 with non-steroidal anti-inflammatory drugs and NSAIDs alone. Osteoarthritis Cartilage 1995;3:213–25.

16. Nallamshetty L, Buchowski JM, Nazarian LA, et al. Septic arthritis of the hip following cortisone injection: case report and review of the literature. Clin Imaging 2003;27(4): 225–8.

17. Chang RW, Pellissier JM, Hazen GB. A cost-effectiveness analysis of total hip arthroplasty for osteoarthritis of the hip. JAMA 1996;275:858–65.

18. Mahomed NN, Barrett JA, Katz JN, et al. Rates and outcomes of primary and revision total hip replacement in the United States Medicare population. J Bone Joint Surg Am 2003;85(1):27–32.

19. Adam RF, Noble J. Primary total knee arthroplasty in the elderly. J Arthroplasty 1994;9:495–7.

20. Bozik KJ, Saleh KJ, Rosenberg AG, et al. Economic evaluation of total hip arthroplasty: analysis and review of the literature. J Arthroplasty 2004;19:180–9.

21. Petersen VS, Solgaard S, Simonsen B. Total hip replacement in patients aged 80 years and older. J Am Geriatr Soc 1989;37:219–22.

22. Brander AB, Malhotra S, Jet J, et al. Outcome of hip and knee arthroplasty in persons aged 80 years and older. Clin Orthop 1997;345:67–78.

23. Hernandez-Vaquero D, Fernandez-Carreira JM, Perez-Hernandez D, et al. Total knee arthroplasty in the elderly. Is there an age limit? J Arthroplasty 2006;21:358–61.

24. Biau D, Mullins MM, Judet T. Is anyone too old for a total knee replacement? Clin Orthop 2006;448:180–4.

25. Karuppiah SV, Banaszkiewicz PA, Ledingham WM. The mortality, morbidity and cost benefits of elective total knee arthroplasty in the nonagenarian population. Int Orthop 2008;32:339–43.

26. Zicat B, Rorabeck CH, Bourne RB, et al. Total knee arthroplasty in the octogenarian. J Arthroplasty 1993;8:395–400.

27. Hosick WB, Lotke PA, Baldwin A. Total knee arthroplasty in patients 80 years of age and older. Clin Orthop 1994;299:77–80.

28. Pettine KA, Aamlid BC, Cabanela ME. Elective Total hip arthroplasty in patients older than 80 years of age. Clin Orthop 1991;266:127–32.

29. Berry DJ, von Knoch M, Schleck CD et al. The cumulative long-term risk of dislocation after primary Charnley total hip arthroplasty. J Bone Joint Surg Am 2004;86(1):9–14.

30. Phillips CB, Barrett JA, Losina E, et al. Incidence rates of dislocation, pulmonary embolism and deep infection during the first 6 months after elective total hip replacement. J Bone Joint Surg Am 2003;85:20–6.

31. Mraovic B, Hipszer BR, Epstein RH, et al. Preadmission hyperglycemia is an independent risk factor for in-hospital symptomatic pulmonary embolism after major orthopedic surgery. J Arthroplasty 2010;25:64–70.

32. Marchant MH, Niens NA, Cook C, et al. The impact of glycemic control and diabetes mellitus on perioperative outcomes after total joint arthroplasty. J Bone Joint Surg Am 2009;91:1621–9.

33. Lieberman JR, Fuchs MD, Haas SB, et al. Hip arthroplasty in patients with chronic renal failure. J Arthroplasty 1995;10(2):191–5.

34. Mantilla CB, Horlocker TT, Schroeder DR, et al. Frequency of myocardial infarction, pulmonary embolism, deep venous thrombosis and death following primary hip or knee arthroplasty. Anesthesiology 2002;96(5):1140–6.

35. Camberlin C, Vrijens F, De Gauguier K, et al. Provider volume and short term complications after elective total hip replacement: an analysis of Belgian administrative data. Acta Orthop Belg 2011;77:311–9.

36. Singh JA, Kwoh CK, Boudreau RM, et al. Hospital volume and surgical outcomes after elective hip/knee arthroplasty. Arthritis Rheum 2011;63:2531–9.

37. Katz JN, Barrett J, Mohomed NN, et al. Association between hospital and surgeon procedure volume and the outcomes of total knee replacement. J Bone Joint Surg Am 2004;86:1909–16.

38. Katz JN, Losina E, Barrett J, et al. Association between hospital and procedure volume and outcomes of total hip replacement in the United States Medicare population. J Bone Joint Surg Am 2001;83:1622–9.

39. Lee J, Singletary R, Schmader K, et al. Surgical site infection in the elderly following orthopaedic surgery, risk factors and outcomes. J Bone Joint Surg. 2006;88:1705–12.

40. Kurtz SM, Ong KL, Lau E, et al. Prosthetic joint infection risk after TKA in the Medicare population. Clin Orthop 2010 468:52–6.

41. Leone JM, Hanssen AD. Management of infection at the site of a total knee arthroplasty. J Bone Joint Surg Am 2005;87:2335–48.

42. Peersman G, Laskin R, Davis G, et al. Infection in knee replacement: a retrospective review of 6489 total knee replacements. Clin Orthop 2001;392:15–23.

43. Pulido L, Ghanem E, Joshi A, et al. Periprosthetic joint infection: the incidence, timing and predisposing factors. Clin Orthop 2008;466(7):1710–5.

44. Patel VP, Walsh M, Sehgal B, et al. Factors associated with prolonged wound drainage after primary total hip and knee arthroplasty. J Bone Joint Surg Am 2007;89(1):33–8.

45. Jamsen E, Huhtala H, Puolakka T, et al. Risk factors for infection after knee arthroplasty, a register-based analysis of 43,149 cases. J Bone Join Surg Am 2009;91(1): 38–47.

46. Kim DH, Spencer M, Davidson SM, et al. Institutional prescreening for detection and eradication of Methicillin-resistant Staphylococcus aureus in patients undergoing elective orthopedic surgery. J Bone Joint Surg Am 2010;92(9):1820–6.

47. Garvin KL, Konigsberg BS. Infection following total knee arthroplasty, prevention and management. J Bone Joint Surg Am 2011;93:1167–75.

48. Spangehl MS, Masri BA, O'Connell JX, et al. Prospective analysis of preoperative and intraoperative investigations for the diagnosis of infection at the site of 202 revision total hip arthroplasty. J Bone Joint Surg Am 1999;81(5):672–83.

49. Ghanem E, Parvizi J, Burnett RS, et al. Cell count and differential of aspirated fluid in the diagnosis of infection at the site of total knee arthroplasty. J Bone Joint Surg Am 2008;90(8):1637–43.

50. Lieberman JR, Hsu WK. Prevention of venous thromboembolic disease after total hip and knee arthroplasty. J Bone Joint Surg Am 2005;87:2097–112.

51. Johanson NA, Lachiewicz PF, Lieberman JR, et al. Prevention of symptomatic pulmonary embolism in patients undergoing total hip or knee arthroplasty. J Am Acad Orthop Surg 2009;17(3):183–96.

52. Bern M, Deshmukh RV, Nelson R, et al. Low-dose warfarin coupled with lower leg compression is effective prophylaxis against thromboembolic disease after hip arthroplasty. J Arthroplasty 2007;644–50.

53. Inouye SK. Delerium in older persons. N Engl J Med 2006;354:1157–65.

54. Robinson TN, Raeburn CD, Tran ZV, et al. Postoperative delirium in the elderly: risk factors and outcomes. Ann Surg 2009;249:173–8.

55. Sampson EL, Raven PR, Ndhlovu PN, et al. A randomized, double-blind, placebo-controlled trial of donepezil hydrochloride (Aricept) for reducing the incidence of postoperative delirium after elective total hip replacement. Int J Geriatr Psychiatry 2007;22:343–9.

56. Larsen KA, Kelly SE, Stern TA, et al. Administration of olanzapine to prevent postoperative delirium in the elderly joint-replacement patient: a randomized controlled trial. Psychosomatics 2010;51:409–18.

57. Leslie DL, Marcantonio ER, Zhang Y, et al. One-year health care costs associated with delirium in the elderly population. Arch Intern Med 2008;168:27–32.

58. Mitchell PA, Greidanus NV, Masri BA, et al. The prevention of periprosthetic fractures of the femur during and after total hip arthroplasty. Instr Course Lect 2003;52:301–8.

59. Bethea JS, DeAndrade JR, Fleming LL, et al. Proximal femoral fractures following total hip arthroplasty. Clin Orthop 1982;170:95–106.

60. Fitzgerald RH, Brindley GW, Kavanagh BF. The uncemented total hip arthroplasty: intraoperative femoral fractures. Clin Orthop 1988;235:61–6.

61. Haddad FS, Masri BA, Garbuz DS, et al. The prevention of periprosthetic fractures in total hip and knee arthroplasty. Orthop Clin North Am 1999;30:191–207.

62. Pellicci PM, Inglis AE, Salvati EA. Perforation of the femoral shaft during total hip replacement, report of twelve cases. J Bone Joint Surg Am 1980;62:234–40.

63. Morrey BF, Kavanagh BF. Complications with revision of the femoral component of total hip arthroplasty, comparison between cemented and uncemented techniques. J Arthroplasty 1992;7:71–9.

64. Berry DJ. Epidemiology. Hip and knee. Orthop Clin North Am 1999;30:183–90.

65. Meek RM, Garbuz DS, Masri BA, et al. Intraoperative fracture of the femur in revision total hip arthroplasty with a diaphyseal fitting stem. J Bone Joint Surg Am 2004;86: 480–5.

66. Somers JF, Suy R, Stuyck J, et al. Conservative treatment of femoral shaft fractures in patients with total hip arthroplasty. J Arthroplasty 1998;13:162–71.

67. Bhattacharya T, Chang D, Meigo JB, et al. Mortality after periprosthetic fracture of the femur. J Bone Joint Surg Am 2007;89(12):2658–62.

68. Berry DJ, von Knoch M, Schleck CD, et al. The cumulative long-term risk of dislocation after primary total hip arthroplasty. J Bone Joint Surg Am 2004;86:9–14.

69. Parvizi J, Picinic E, Sharkey PF. Revision total hip arthroplasty for instability: surgical techniques and principles. J Bone Joint Surg Am 2008;90:1134–42.

70. Von Knocch M, Berry DJ, Harmsen WS, et al. Late dislocation after total hip arthroplasty. J Bone Joint Surg Am 2002;84:1949–53.

71. Paterno SA, Lachiewicz PF, Kelley SS. The influence of patient-related factors and the position of the acetabular component on the rate of dislocation after total hip replacement. J Bone Joint Surg Am 1997;79:1202–10.

72. Daly PJ, Morrey BF. Operative correction of an unstable total hip arthroplasty. J Bone Joint Surg Am 1992;74:1334–42.
73. Parvizi J, Mui A, Purtill JJ, et al. Total joint arthroplasty: when do fatal or near-fatal complications occur. J Bone Joint Surg Am 2007;89:27–32.
74. Pulido L, Parvizi J, Macgibeny M, et al. In hospital complications after total joint replacement. J Arthroplasty 2008;23(6 Suppl 1):139–45.
75. Mortazavi SM, Kakli H, Orhan B, et al. Perioperative stroke after total joint arthroplasty: prevalence, predictors and outcome. J Bone Joint Surg Am 2010;92:2095–101.
76. Basilico F, Sweeney G, Losina E, et al. Risk factors for cardiovascular complications following total joint replacement surgery. Arthritis Rheum 2008;58:1915–20.
77. Parvizi J, Pulido L, Slenker N, et al. Vascular injuries after total joint arthroplasty. J Arthroplasty 2008;23:1115–21.
78. Calligaro KD, Dougherty MJ, Ryan S, et al. Acute arterial complications associated with total hip and knee arthroplasty. J Vasc Surg 2003;38:1170–7.
79. Farrell CM, Springer BD, Haidukewych GJ, et al. Motor nerve palsy following primary total hip arthroplasty. J Bone Joint Surg Am 2005;87:2619–25.
80. DeHart MM, Riley LH. Nerve injuries in total hip arthroplasty. J Am Acad Orthop Surg 1999;7(2):101–11.
81. Schinsky MF, Macaulay W, Parks ML, et al. Nerve injury after primary total knee arthroplasty. J Arthroplasty 2001;16:1048–54.
82. Krackow KA, Maar DC, Mont MA, et al. Surgical decompression for peroneal nerve palsy after total knee arthroplasty. Clin Orthop 1993;292:223.

Rehabilitation and Total Joint Arthroplasty

Marie D. Westby, BSc (PT), PhD[a,b,*]

KEYWORDS

- Total joint arthroplasty • Rehabilitation • Physical therapy • Older adults

KEY POINTS

- Older adults experience numerous benefits from total joint arthroplasty (TJA); however, rehabilitation goals, approaches, and duration may differ for geriatric patients with additional age-related musculoskeletal, cognitive, and sensory impairments.
- The rehabilitation plan should address patients' needs along the TJA continuum from preoperative through the postacute phase and return to independence in activities of daily living, mobility, and valued leisure and sporting activities.
- Progressive resistance training with sufficient intensity and dosage to enable a physiologic training effect should be a key component of any rehabilitation program.
- Both individual and group exercise programs can be beneficial, and the level of health professional supervision should be matched to the patient's needs.
- It is important to educate and encourage patients to become more physically active following TJA surgery in order to achieve health-enhancing benefits associated with regular moderate-intensity exercise.
- Recovery after total knee arthroplasty is longer than after total hip arthroplasty and requires a longer period of supervised rehabilitation for optimal outcomes.
- A variety of contextual factors including a patient's coping skills, self-efficacy, anxiety, and social support are associated with perceived well-being and satisfaction after TJA surgery and therefore should be identified and addressed in the perioperative period.

INTRODUCTION

More than 77,000 Canadians underwent total hip arthroplasty (THA) and total knee arthroplasty (TKA) surgeries in 2008 and 2009[1] and more than 10 times this number in the United States.[2] By far the majority of patients undergoing these elective procedures are in the 65 to 74 years age group. However, there has been a significant

The author has nothing to disclose.
[a] Mary Pack Arthritis Program, 895 West 10th Avenue, Vancouver, BC V5Z 1L7, Canada;
[b] Department of Physical Therapy, University of British Columbia, 212-2177 Wesbrook Mall, Vancouver, BC V6T 1Z3, Canada
* 895 West 10th Avenue, Vancouver, BC, V5Z 1L7 Canada.
E-mail address: Marie.westby@vch.ca

rise in number of surgeries in the 75 years and older cohort with increases of 65% and 122% over the past decade for THA and TKA procedures, respectively.[1] Osteoarthritis (OA) is the primary diagnosis leading to total joint arthroplasty (TJA) and contributes to 81% of THA and 94% of TKA surgeries.[1] With the aging of the North American population and the alarmingly higher prevalence of obesity and inactivity, it is not surprising that the annual number of THA and TKA surgeries is projected to jump to more than 4 million in the United States[3] by the year 2030. These high-volume surgical procedures and accompanying rehabilitation interventions will have increasingly greater impacts on health care systems and resource allocation for rehabilitation services.[4-6]

Much attention has been directed at addressing lengthy wait times and reducing acute care length of stay (LOS) for THA and TKA surgery in Canada[1,7] and other countries. Conversely, little research and resources have been allocated to evaluating cost-effective TJA rehabilitation.[8] Despite being an understudied aspect of the TJA surgical continuum, an increasing body of evidence is available to inform rehabilitation practices.

CURRENT STATE OF TJA REHABILITATION

According to the World Health Organization, "Rehabilitation is a process aimed at enabling individuals to reach and maintain their optimal physical, sensory, intellectual, psychological, and social functional levels."[9] Rehabilitation involves contributions from many health disciplines including physical therapy and occupational therapy and is offered in a variety of inpatient, outpatient, and community settings. In TJA, rehabilitation may include education and exercise interventions prior to surgery, early mobilization during the short acute care stay, and exercise, gait, and balance training postoperatively.[10] However, current approaches to TJA rehabilitation vary greatly at local, national, and international levels.[11-14] The inconsistencies extend to specific therapeutic interventions, outcome evaluation, and follow-up care,[11,13,15] and practice variation can only be partially explained by patient factors.

Efforts are under way in Canada,[16,17] including the author's own, and abroad[18-20] to improve the consistency and quality of TJA surgical and rehabilitation care. For example, Bone and Joint Canada has developed an online toolkit that includes recommendations for components of a National Core Model of Care for primary hip and knee replacement surgery and resources addressing wait times and preoperative, surgical, and postoperative care and evaluation.[17] Yet to date, no evidence-based clinical practice guidelines with detailed recommendations are available in North America to help clinicians and patients make informed decisions about appropriate rehabilitation care.

FUNCTIONAL RECOVERY AFTER TJA

Prospective, observational studies have increased our understanding of "typical" functional recovery after THA and TKA. The greatest functional gains take place during the first 6 months after THA[21-23] and within 12 months after TKA,[21,22] with self-reported function improving earlier and more so than performance-based tasks.[21,23,24] There is agreement among patients, clinicians, and researchers that individuals undergoing TKA recover function at a slower rate and to a lesser extent than THA[21,22,25,26] and require more postoperative rehabilitation.[7,26] Bourne and colleagues[26] compared primary THA and TKA patient outcomes in 3050 patients 1 year postsurgery and found that a higher percentage of patients with a THA indicated they would have their surgery again (96%) compared with those with TKA (89%), and self-reported function and overall satisfaction with pain and function were also better among patients with a THA.[26] Primary (first time) procedures are associated with fewer perioperative complications and readmissions and greater functional recovery than revision surgeries.[27] Patients with inflammatory arthritis such as rheumatoid arthritis have greater complication rates and less favorable outcomes than those with OA,[28] although they too experience marked benefits with TJA surgery.[29] This article focuses on primary TJA for OA.

Postoperative Pain

Whereas patients can anticipate good to excellent pain reduction, physical function, and health-related quality of life (HRQoL) following TJA surgery,[30–32] as much as 25% of patients report protracted postsurgical pain, functional impairments, and activity limitations more than 2 years after surgery.[24,33–36] At 7-year follow-up, about 20% of patients would not undergo the procedure again because of difficult recovery or unsatisfactory results.[37] Unsatisfactory pain levels are especially evident following TKA.[38] Protracted pain may be due to the surgery itself (eg, failing components, infection, malposition) or due to musculoskeletal causes including degenerative changes in the lumbar spine or hip.[39–41] In a prospective follow-up study of 83 patients with a mean age of 66 years, greater post-TKA pain at 1 year was related to preoperative pain levels, anxiety, and depression.[42]

Postoperative Impairment

Postoperative impairments in muscle strength and activation are most evident in the first month following TKA and slowly recover to only slightly better than presurgical levels between 6 and 12 months post surgery.[24] On average, patients with a unilateral TKA exhibit quadriceps strength deficits of between 12% and 31% compared with the nonoperated side and 34% to 37% compared with that of age and gender-matched peers as much as 13 years after surgery.[24] Similar protracted muscle weakness is reported for the hip abductors following THA.[39,43,44] At the knee, quadriceps weakness is believed to be a result of both muscle atrophy and neuromuscular activation (muscle inhibition) deficits.[24,45] Other impairments contributing to delayed and sometimes incomplete functional recovery after THA and TKA include muscle contractures,[39] limb length differences,[39,46] malalignment,[39] balance deficits,[47] and functional limitations in gait[34,48] and more complex tasks such as climbing stairs.[49,50] In a 12-month prospective follow-up study of 8050 patients who underwent primary TKA, 31% reported little or no improvement in physical function as measured by the short form–12 (SF-12).[51] It is estimated that only about 40% of the functional limitations present at least 1 year after TKA are attributable to the normal physiologic effects of aging.[50] These combined strength and functional limitations put individuals at increased risk of falls and reduced functional independence.[52]

Postoperative Activity

Physical inactivity among older adults and individuals with arthritis is a major public health concern.[53,54] Physical activity levels following TJA have primarily been assessed through questionnaires involving patient recall of past or current physical activity, and increasingly more often through motion sensors (pedometer, accelerometer). There have been mixed findings with self-report questionnaires tending to overestimate actual activity levels. Instrumented assessment suggests that individuals with a primary THA reach population norms with respect to level of physical activity.[55] Being younger (<65 years) and male are associated with greater levels of

---

Box 1
Considerations for rehabilitation providers working with elderly TJA patients

- Increased risk for falls and related fractures
- Marked reductions in muscle mass and strength
- Decreased soft tissue and joint flexibility
- Reduced functional aerobic capacity
- Cognitive and sensory impairments
- Greater likelihood of significant comorbidities and postsurgical adverse events
- More likely to live alone or require social support

---

physical activity.[55] Over the first year following TKA surgery, patients expend similar levels of energy as they did preoperatively; however, the amount of time spent walking remains below age-matched healthy controls.[56] Being younger, male, less overweight, and more physically active preoperatively were associated with greater physical activity levels and sports participation through a retrospective chart review of 736 patients 1 year following TJA.[57] Although some studies show health-enhancing physical activity levels approaching population norms, they also reveal that a large percentage of patients are not physically active enough[58] and have not adopted a more active lifestyle after TJA surgery.[56] This result is despite evidence to suggest that individuals with higher lifelong physical activity levels achieve greater functional scores 4 years after a TKA.[59] It is important to educate and encourage patients to become or remain physically active after TJA surgery to improve general health and HRQoL and maintain musculoskeletal function and the ability to live independently.[53]

Postoperative Participation

Participation in social and leisure activities and return to valued life roles including paid work have been less studied in the TJA population yet are expressed concerns of both younger and older patients within the first few months after surgery.[16,22,60,61] HRQoL is a complex, multifaceted construct that has most often been measured through the short form–36 (SF-36) questionnaire and its shortened version, the SF-12, following TJA.[30] Significant improvements in HRQoL take place in the 12 months following THA and TKA surgery.[30,62] However, as many as 1 in 2 patients do not reach HRQoL levels of the age-standardized general population.[62] Further, approximately one-quarter of patients are unable to perform their valued leisure activities 1 year after TJA surgery.[38]

Elderly patients face additional challenges to full recovery along the TJA continuum that rehabilitation providers need to take into consideration (see **Box 1**). These challenges may include increased risk for postsurgical adverse events,[63,64] longer acute care LOS,[64] musculoskeletal impairments (eg, sarcopenia, osteopenia/osteoporosis),[65] cognitive challenges (short term memory loss),[66] sensory impairments (hearing, visual), comorbidities, sleep issues,[16] and changes in living situation and social support. However, older age alone is not associated with worse clinical outcomes[67] or longer recovery after TJA surgery.[68] Frailty is more of an issue than age alone. Sarcopenia, a progressive reduction in skeletal muscle mass, strength, and quality, is often observed with aging.[69] This condition greatly contributes to frailty in older adults and results in reduced physical performance, endurance, and resistance capacity and increased risk of falls and fractures.[70] The combined impact is a loss of independence, which is a concern expressed by many individuals undergoing TJA.[16]

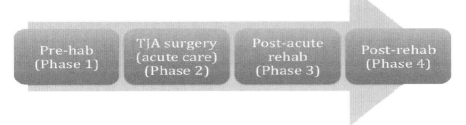

Fig. 1. The TJA rehabilitation continuum.

THE TJA CONTINUUM

There is growing appreciation for conceptualizing TJA rehabilitation on a continuum and identifying an individual's health and psychosocial needs along this trajectory (**Fig. 1**). The TJA continuum can be broken down into four phases: "pre-hab," acute, postacute, and post rehab; although terms and time frames used to describe these stages may differ. Once TJA surgery is identified as a viable option, the individual should be considered "on the continuum."

Phase 1: Pre-Hab

The pre-habilitation or pre-hab phase extends from the point at which an individual is deemed a candidate for THA or TKA surgery to the day of surgery. In some parts of the world including Canada, this period is often more than 6 months,[71,72] whereas in the United States, wait times are much shorter,[73] and the time available to participate in pre-hab is limited. During this phase there is an opportunity to minimize the functional decline and reduction in HRQoL reported by individuals awaiting TJA surgery.[74,75] Ideally, individuals living with hip or knee OA are already participating in a regular self-management and exercise program that addresses physical and psychosocial needs, thus maintaining function, activity, and participation during the course of their OA. The roles of pre-hab would then simply be to prepare for surgery through (1) education about the surgical procedure (eg, complications), postoperative recovery, and rehabilitation; (2) preparation of the home environment and arrangements for social support; (3) prescription and instruction on use of walking aid; (4) addressing medical issues and lifestyle factors that may adversely impact surgical outcome (eg, smoking, nutrition); and (5) modification of the exercise program to best address the physical demands inherent with undergoing a major orthopaedic procedure (eg, upper limb strength training to prepare for use of walking aids and transfers).[17,76] Studies show, however, that less than 30% of persons with physician-diagnosed arthritis participate in moderate physical activity and exercise that meets current guidelines for health,[54] and those awaiting TJA surgery are markedly deconditioned.[77]

As a result, this preoperative phase provides an opportunity to introduce appropriate exercise, address barriers to exercise behaviors, and promote a physically active lifestyle after surgery. The effects of preoperative education, exercise, and behavioral interventions have been studied in individuals awaiting TJA. Comprehensive education prior to surgery allows patients and their families to prepare for the surgical and rehabilitation experience and become engaged in the process.[76] It is recommended that health professionals use a variety of educational methods including print, audiovisual, and interactive sessions that allow patients and families to ask questions and address their individual needs.[17,76] In a Cochrane review on the effects of preoperative education within 6 weeks of TKA or THA, results showed a modest positive effect on preoperative anxiety; however, no effect on pain, functioning, acute care LOS, or postoperative anxiety.[78] Such findings suggest that education alone, through written, verbal, or audiovisual formats, is insufficient in preparing patients and that patients may need more time to incorporate the information. Furthermore, there may be patient subgroups that are more likely to respond favorably to specific educational interventions.

Most patients will also benefit from preoperative conditioning and guidance on how to remain physically active prior to surgery. Whereas this regimen can be a challenge for the person with tremendous pain and marked activity limitations associated with end-stage hip and knee OA, it remains an important goal. In a qualitative study examining patients and health provider views on TJA rehabilitation, the overwhelming advice from patients was to take an active role in the preparation for and recovery from surgery, which included doing as much exercise as possible prior to the TJA.[16] In a systematic review of English language articles published prior to August 2003, Ackerman and Bennell[79] reported on five controlled trials examining the effects of a preoperative exercise or physical therapy program. Significant and small to moderate improvements were found for self-reported function, hip flexion range of motion (ROM), hip strength, and varied gait parameters at 12 and 24 weeks after THA surgery; however, the two included studies reporting on the same patient cohort also included postoperative exercise therapy, which confounds the results. From the three TKA studies, the investigators concluded that small treatment effects in self-reported function, knee ROM, knee strength, and walking speed resulted from preoperative exercise interventions delivered over 5- or 6-week periods.[74] In a more recent review of trials published up to January 2006, developers from the French Physical Medicine and Rehabilitation Society's guideline development program reported on the heterogeneous nature of the preoperative interventions, and despite the shortcomings of the available evidence, recommended a multidisciplinary rehabilitation program composed of at least occupational therapy and education to the most fragile patients with major disability, comorbidity, or limited social support.[80] Trials published subsequent to these reviews have reported beneficial functional outcomes following pre-THA and TKA land-based and pool-based exercise programs[81] and a partially supervised strengthening and aerobic exercise program performed three times a week within 4 weeks of TKA surgery.[82] Even greater benefits can be achieved if this latter progressive pre-hab exercise program is started earlier and carried out over a 4- to 8-week period prior to surgery.[69,83]

Cognitive behavior interventions aimed at improving anxiety, coping, and self-efficacy have also been studied during the preoperative phase. Daltroy and colleagues[84] observed that greater preoperative anxiety and depression resulted in poorer outcomes after TJA and conducted a randomized controlled trial (RCT) with 222 elderly patients undergoing THA or TKA to examine the effects of relaxation training provided the day prior to surgery.[84] Patients who exhibited the most denial had significantly shorter acute LOS and less pain medication use, whereas those with greater baseline anxiety experienced less postoperative anxiety with the relaxation intervention. There was no effect on postoperative pain, which the investigators attributed to insufficient time to practice the relaxation response and poor adherence to the regimen. It is important to assess and attend to the patient's psychological state and level of preparation prior to surgery and, where appropriate, include strategies such as calming self-talk, mental relaxation, and cognitive restructuring techniques to improve coping and other psychological outcomes.[84,85]

Phase 2: Acute Care

The acute care stay is characterized by increasingly shorter LOS during which any meaningful rehabilitation can be initiated. However, with the implementation of clinical pathways over the past 30 years, there have been improvements in the quality of inpatient acute care provided after TJA with significant reductions in postoperative complications[20] and hospital costs and more patients being discharged to home, as well as shorter LOS.[20,86] Common to most pathways is the emphasis on early mobilization,[13] which is usually initiated the day following surgery.[87–89] Additional early rehabilitation goals during this stage include pain management, prophylactic thromboembolitic therapy, addressing perioperative complications (eg, postanaesthetic delirium, anemia), bowel and bladder function, transfer training, independence in self-care, and discharge planning. Daily physical therapy is recommended.[17,87,89]

Phase 3: Postacute Rehabilitation

The majority of rehabilitation takes place during the postacute phase once a patient has been discharged from the acute care setting. Systematic reviews examining multidisciplinary rehabilitation[90] and physical therapy or exercise interventions after TJA[18,19,91–94] have concluded that small to moderate benefits in lower limb muscle strength and function are achieved in the short term. However, most differences between supervised exercise and unsupervised exercise or alternate therapy groups have disappeared by 1-year follow-up. A summary of systematic reviews evaluating the effects of varied rehabilitation interventions after THA and TKA and controlled trials published since the reviews is provided in **Table 1**.

Considerations when designing an individualized postacute rehabilitation program include setting (outpatient, inpatient, or home-based), timing (immediately after discharge from acute hospital setting or delayed by several weeks for THA patients), level of supervision (1:1 vs group care), and type of program (land-based or pool-based). In a primarily white, female sample of more than 164,000 individuals from four states in the United States, 55% of patients were discharged home, and of these, 58% received home health care.[14] Of those discharged to an inpatient facility, 65% received care at a specialized nursing facility, whereas the remainder received their rehabilitation in an inpatient rehabilitation facility. Among other variables, older individuals were more likely to receive inpatient or institutional care.[14] The authors of a systematic review of acute and postacute rehabilitation following THA found that interventions commenced within a month of surgery were more likely to be beneficial if performed in an outpatient center.[94] There have been no head-to-head comparisons of identical rehabilitation programs (eg, same level of supervision, therapeutic protocol, equipment) being provided in an outpatient setting compared with a patient's home. Rather, investigators have drawn conclusions about the appropriateness of a given setting based on studies with confounding factors such as different rehabilitation formats and levels of supervision that likely contributed to the intervention's effectiveness.[97,98]

The timing of rehabilitation is believed to be more critical following TKA surgery; however, rehabilitation initiated early in the postoperative period is recommended for both surgeries.[94] An Austrian study compared the effects of a 4-week inpatient rehabilitation program delivered at three different time periods following cementless THA surgery and concluded that early intervention (provided within 2 months of surgery) resulted in better walking speed at 12-month follow-up than the same

Table 1
Overview of rehabilitation interventions and clinical outcomes following primary TJA

Study ID	Sample Demographics	Intervention	Control	Outcomes	Results
THA					
Minns Lowe 2009[91] (systematic review)	Eight RCTs (n = 282) of patients with hip OA, no mean ages provided.	Various outpatient and home-based exercise programs, individual and group supervision, duration ranged from 5 to 15 weeks, frequency ranged from daily to 1–4 days/week.	Usual or standard care or comparison of two different types of physiotherapy intervention.	Functional ADL, walking, HRQoL, muscle strength and hip ROM.	Significant benefits for walking speed and hip abductor strength. Metaanalysis not appropriate for other outcomes. Mixed results and poor trial quality prevented drawing conclusions on effectiveness of posthospital physiotherapy.
Di Monaco 2009[93] (systematic review)	Nine controlled trials (n = 348) of patients with hip OA, mean age ranged from 45 to 75 years.	Various physical exercises performed in hospital or after discharge from hospital, duration ranged from 4 days to 1 year, frequency ranged from daily to 3 days/week.	Standard care or comparison of two different types of exercise intervention.	At least 1 among impairment, activity, HRQoL, or hospital LOS.	Convincing evidence for effectiveness of treadmill training, unilateral resistance training, and arm-ergometry exercises in addition to standard exercise. Late exercise (>8 weeks post-op) is useful if it includes weight-bearing exercise and hip abductor strengthening.
Okoro 2012[94] (systematic review)	Eleven RCTs (n = 986) of patients with hip OA, no mean ages provided.	Various inpatient acute, outpatient and home-based rehabilitation interventions, duration ranged from 1 to 12 weeks, frequency ranged from daily to 2 days/week.	Not specified.	Functional outcome and dislocation rate.	Early interventions (≤1 month post-THA) resulted in statistically significant functional benefits if center-based and included progressive resistance training. Late (>1 month post-THA) home-based interventions led to significant short-term functional improvements.

TKA

Study	Design/Population	Intervention	Comparison	Outcomes	Results
Minns Lowe 2007[92] (systematic review)	Six RCTs (n = 614) of patients with knee OA, no mean ages provided.	Various outpatient and home-based exercise programs, individual and group supervision, duration ranged from 3 to 10 weeks, frequency ranged from 2 to 7 days/week.	Usual or standard care or comparison of two different types of physiotherapy intervention.	Self-reported function, walking speed, ROM, HRQoL, muscle strength.	Small to moderate effect sizes favoring functional exercise for short-term self-reported function and ROM. No long-term benefit.
Petterson 2009[95] (RCT)	Two treatment arms (n = 200) of patients with knee OA, mean age 65 years, 46% female.	EG 1: progressive LE strength training on outpatient setting; 2 to 3 days/week for 6 weeks.	EG 2: same exercise program + neuromuscular electrical stimulation to quadriceps while performing 10 isokinetic quadriceps contractions.	Volitional isometric contraction, timed up & go, stair climbing test, 6 min walk test.	No significant between-group differences in any short- or long-term outcomes. Progressive quadriceps strengthening with or without neuromuscular electrical stimulation enhances clinical improvement after TKA.
Harmer 2009[96] (RCT)	Two treatment arms (n = 102) of patients with knee OA, mean age 68 years, 57% female.	EG 1: land-based group exercise program in outpatient setting; 2 days/week for 6 weeks.	EG 2: pool-based group exercise in community pool; 2 days/week for 6 weeks.	6 min walk test, stair climbing power, WOMAC, ROM.	Significant improvements in all outcomes for both groups at 8 weeks and 6-month follow-up with no between-group differences.

Abbreviations: ADL, activities of daily living; EG, experimental group; LE, lower extremity; WOMAC, Western Ontario McMaster University Osteoarthritis Index.

program at 3 to 4 and 11 months postsurgery.[99] Yet, the evidence also shows beneficial effects on function and balance from late-phase exercise programs provided between 8 and 12 months[100] and 1.5 years after THA[101] and on muscle strength, function, and mobility as much as 4 years following TKA.[102] A recent RCT from Germany compared the effects of early (6 days postoperative) and late (14 days postoperative) aquatic exercise therapy after TKA and THA on self-reported function, HRQoL, and patient satisfaction.[103] There were no significant between-group differences in any of the outcomes in the short or long term; however, earlier aquatic exercise favored individuals with a TKA whereas later participation favored those with a THA.

The level of rehabilitation provider supervision was examined through a sequential cohort study comparing a circuit-based group exercise program delivered in an outpatient setting twice a week to a home-based individualized therapy program with a physical therapist (PT) visit once a week. Despite more variables than level of supervision being examined in this study design (ie, setting and treatment frequency), the investigators found no difference between the two groups for self-reported and performance-based function, HRQoL, and ROM, with both groups improving over a 12-week period, and concluded that group-based exercise was the more efficient method of delivery.[97] Naylor and colleagues[104] explored patient preference for individual and group-based therapy after TKA by surveying 93 subjects 1 year following surgery. They found that most patients were highly satisfied with their mode of rehabilitation, and no overall preference for one mode emerged. The most common reasons for preferring individual therapy were greater guidance and a personalized approach, whereas for group-based therapy, the opportunity to compare progress and social/peer support was cited.[104]

In a large RCT comparing the effects of a PT-led group land-based exercise program to a PT-led group pool program over a 6-week period after TKA surgery, similar short- and long-term benefits were found for pain relief, self-reported function, mobility, and stair-climbing power.[96] Both land-based and pool-based exercise result in meaningful improvements in patient functioning and similar levels of patient satisfaction.

Although no one rehabilitation approach or therapeutic intervention has been judged superior to another, researchers, clinicians, and patients are in agreement that health professional–supervised, functional exercise programs that are regularly progressed are needed to optimize patient outcomes.[52,94] Basic ROM and low-intensity strengthening exercises, traditionally prescribed during the acute care phase, are less effective.[94,100] A phased exercise program with progression of low-intensity exercises prescribed during the acute phase to more intensive resistance training, weightbearing, and advanced functional exercises is most appropriate. Progressive resistance training, which challenges the skeletal muscles with loads that can be repeatedly lifted (8 to 15 repetitions) before the onset of neuromuscular fatigue, are recommended.[94,105] Further, to promote physiologic adaptation, the training load and/or volume need to be progressed on a regular basis.[106] In a more detailed examination of specific therapeutic exercises in the 4 to 5 months following TKA, Meier and colleagues[24] outlined a four-stage physical therapy program including goals, exercises, gait training, and modalities that progresses from the outpatient or home setting to a community-based gym. Similarly, Bade and Stevens-Lapsley[52] have reported success with a high-intensity rehabilitation program also involving four phases up to 12 weeks post-TKA. This author is not aware of a detailed, phased therapeutic exercise program that has been published for THA.

Individuals who experience delayed or poor functional recovery after TJA may require further clinical examinations and diagnostic procedures. Impairments identified earlier as being linked to poor recovery following THA and TKA[39-41] and including persistent postoperative pain, muscle weakness, soft tissue contractures, leg length discrepancy, malalignment in one or both lower limbs, and mechanical or degenerative problems in other joints, will warrant additional rehabilitation to optimize patient outcomes. Strategies may include knee bracing, shoe lifts, foot orthoses, electrical stimulation, peroneal nerve releases, intramuscular botulinum toxin injections, and corticosteroid injections.[39,107]

Phase 4: Post Rehab

There is growing interest in the role that community-based exercise programs can play in helping individuals further their functional recovery and resumption of physically active lifestyles after TJA. This phase begins once the patient has been discharged from the structured, therapist-supervised rehabilitation program, whether that is a home-based, outpatient, or inpatient intervention. No longer "under the health care umbrella," yet understanding the importance of ongoing exercise and resumption of active and healthy lifestyles, many individuals seek out recreational programs designed for those with arthritis and TJA. Such programs are typically offered at community recreation, fitness, or senior centers on a drop-in or registration basis and may have been developed through national organizations using evidence-based processes[53] or at the local level using less well-described methods. Offerings range from group programs in a pool or dance/fitness studio to individualized personal training sessions in a weight-room setting. The amount and quality of supervision varies with post rehab programs. Some facilities offer participants the expertise and guidance of university-educated exercise professionals (eg, exercise physiologist, kinesiologist), whereas others provide supervision through trained fitness instructors or personal trainers with varying levels of experience and knowledge about TJA and appropriate exercise recommendations (personal observation). A number of evidence-based physical activity programs are available in the Unites States and are recommended for people with arthritis and TJA.[53] The American Council on Exercise (www.acefitness.org) and other national fitness organizations offer online courses and resources on the role of the fitness trainer in the rehabilitation continuum, which include specific exercises and progressions and safety guidelines for clients with TJA.

There is a paucity of published research on the effects of community-based, post rehab programs on functional and physical activity outcomes after TJA. In one trial examining the effectiveness of once-weekly gym-based exercise in older adults, 11 of the 106 study participants had undergone a TJA.[108] However, no subgroup analysis was performed, and therefore no conclusions could be drawn as to the benefits of the gym-based aerobic, resistance, and balance training program for individuals with TJA. No adverse events were reported among any participants. Considerations when selecting a post rehab or other recreational exercise program following TJA are listed in **Table 2**.

FACTORS AFFECTING PATIENT OUTCOMES AFTER TJA

A number of factors are known to influence outcomes after TJA and should be identified and, where possible, addressed prior to surgery. These contextual factors can be categorized using the International Classification of Functioning, Disability and Health (ICF) as personal and environmental factors.[109] Although personal factors have yet to be coded in the ICF framework, several have been explored in patients

Table 2	
Considerations when selecting a community-based exercise program after TJA	
Accessibility	• Accessible building, change rooms, pool. and fitness facilities. • Proximity to public transportation or parking. • Access to trained fitness professionals or appropriate supervision. • Choice of individualized or group programs appropriate for clients with TJA.
Costs	• Reasonable costs with option of only paying for sessions attended. • Ability to observe or participate in a session prior to committing to a membership or program fee.
Quality of instruction or programs	• Instructor(s) has experience and/or specific training in working with individuals with TJA. • Program goals and exercises are appropriate for persons with TJA (eg, evidence-based, low impact, not technically demanding). • Exercises are progressed to meet the changing needs of the client.
Communication and collaboration	• Instructor(s) has established links with a health professional or rehabilitation facility to provide guidance should any concerns arise. • Instructor is willing to collaborate with a client's PT or other health care provider if needed.
Equipment and exercise area	• Facility has good variety of aerobic and resistance training equipment appropriate for use after TJA. • It is easy to initiate and adjust equipment and settings to accommodate individual needs (eg, limited knee flexion). • Equipment is clean and well-maintained. • Uncluttered exercise area that is free of obstacles that may lead to falls.

Modified from Westby MD, Minor MA. Exercise and physical activity. In: Bartlett SJ, Bingham CO, Maricic MJ, et al, editors. Clinical care in the rheumatic diseases. 3rd edition. Atlanta (GA): Association of Rheumatology Health Professionals; 2006. p. 216, with permission.

undergoing TJA surgery. In a review of 8050 charts of patients who had undergone a primary TKA 12 months previously, better physical function, as measured by the SF-12 Physical Component Summary score, was found to be associated with younger age, body mass index less than 40, higher SF-12 Mental Component Summary score, and better quadriceps strength preoperatively.[51] Preoperative pain and functional status as well as a greater number of comorbid conditions are also associated with poorer outcomes after TJA surgery.[31] Additional contextual factors that have been studied and linked to outcomes in this patient population are shown in **Fig. 2**.

Environmental factors associated with TJA outcomes include socioeconomic factors, social support, and provider and system level attributes (eg, volume of surgeries performed by surgeon).[124] In a prospective follow-up study of 241 patients undergoing TKA, lower education level and less tangible social support were associated with worse pain and functional outcomes at 6 months after surgery.[110]

SUMMARY

The long-term outcomes following primary TJA for OA are favorable. However, surgery alone fails to fully restore physical function and address longstanding impairments associated with chronic joint disease. Older adults undergoing TJA can

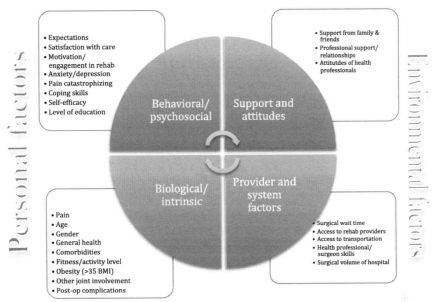

Fig. 2. Contextual factors affecting patient outcomes after primary TJA for OA. (*Data from* Refs.[31,52,62,68,110,111–123])

gain similar benefits as those who are younger; however, the elderly are at increased risk for adverse events. Frailty, more so than age, is related to suboptimal outcomes. To what extent appropriate and sufficient rehabilitation can further improve health outcomes including activity and participation and positively impact prosthesis survival and need for revision is still unclear. There is evidence to suggest that evaluation and management of perioperative psychosocial and other patient factors are important in enhancing outcomes after TJA. Further, there is a growing body of research that points to the importance of progressive resistance training after TJA to address the muscle weakness associated with aging and end-stage hip and knee OA, and secondary to the surgery itself, and to optimize functional outcomes. With the projected increases in number of individuals undergoing TJA over the next two decades, it becomes even more critical to develop cost-effective rehabilitation strategies and identify individuals who would most benefit from such interventions.

REFERENCES

1. Canadian Institute for Health Information. Hip and total knee replacements in Canada—Canadian Joint Replacement Registry. 2008–2009 Annual Report. Available at: www.cihi.ca/cjrr. Accessed September 17, 2009.
2. DeFrances CJ, Lucas CA, Verita CB, et al. 2006 National Hospital Discharge Survey. U.S. Department of Health and Human Services, Centers for Disease Control and Prevention and National Center for Health Statistics; 2008 Jul. Report No. 5. Available at: http://www.cdc.gov/nchs/data/nhsr/nhsr005.pdf. Accessed November 21, 2009.
3. Kurtz S, Ong K, Lau E, et al. Projections of primary and revision hip and knee arthroplasty in the United States from 2005 to 2030. J Bone Joint Surg Am 2007;89(4):780–5.

4. Hawker GA, Badley EM, Croxford R, et al. A population-based nested case-control study of the costs of hip and knee replacement surgery. Med Care 2009;47(97):732–41.
5. Tian W, DeJong G, Brown M, et al. Looking upstream: factors shaping the demand for postacute joint replacement rehabilitation. Arch Phys Med Rehabil 2009;90(8): 1260–8.
6. Antoniou J, Martineau P, Filion K, et al. In-hospital cost of total hip arthroplasty in Canada and the United States. J Bone Joint Surg Am 2004;86–A(11):2435–9.
7. Fancott C, Jaglal S, Quan V, et al. Rehabilitation services following total joint replacement: a qualitative analysis of key processes and structures to decrease length of stay and increase surgical volumes in Ontario, Canada. J Eval Clin Pract 2010;16(4):724–30.
8. National Institutes of Health. NIH consensus development conference on total knee replacement. NIH Consens State Sci Statements 2003 Dec 8–10;20(1):1–34. Available at: http://consensus.hin.gov/2003/2003TotalKneeReplacement117PDF.pdf. Accessed March 17, 2004.
9. World Health Organization. Health topics: rehabilitation. Available at: http://www.who.int/topics/rehabilitation/en/. Accessed October 11, 2011.
10. Ganz SB, Viellion G. Pre and post surgical management of the hip and knee. In: Wegener ST, Belza BL, Gall EP, editors. Clinical care in the rheumatic diseases. Atlanta (GA): American College of Rheumatology; 1996. p. 103–6.
11. Lingard EA, Berven S, Katz JN, et al. Management and care of patients undergoing total knee arthroplasty: variations across different health care settings. Arthritis Care Res 2000;13(3):129–36.
12. Mahomed NN, Lau JT, Lin MK, et al. Significant variation exists in home care services following total joint arthroplasty. J Rheumatol 2004;31(5):973–5.
13. Roos EM. Effectiveness and practice variation of rehabilitation after joint replacement. Curr Opin Rheumatol 2003;15(2):160–2.
14. Freburger JK, Holmes GM, Ku LJ, et al. Disparities in post–acute rehabilitation care for joint replacement. Arthritis Care Res 2011;63(7):1020–30.
15. Naylor J, Harmer A, Fransen M, et al. Status of physiotherapy rehabilitation after total knee replacement in Australia. Phys Res Int 2006;11(1):35–47.
16. Westby MD, Backman CL. Patient and health professional views on rehabilitation practices and outcomes following total hip and knee arthroplasty: a focus group study. BMC Health Services Research 2010;10:119. Available at: http://www.biomedcentral.com.ezproxy.library.ubc.ca/1472-6963/10/119. Accessed December 15, 2011.
17. Waddell JP, Frank C. Hip and knee replacement toolkit, Bone and Joint Canada. Updated March 31, 2011. Available at: www.boneandjointcanada.com. Accessed December 15, 2011.
18. Genêt F, Gouin F, Coudeyre E, et al. The benefits of ambulatory physiotherapy after total hip replacement. Clinical practice recommendations. Ann Readapt Med Phys 2007;50(9):776–82.
19. Genêt F, Mascard E, Coudeyre E, et al. The benefits of ambulatory physiotherapy after total knee replacement. Clinical practice recommendations. Ann Readapt Med Phys 2007;50(9):793–801.
20. Swierstra BA, Vervest AM, Walenkamp GH, et al. Dutch guideline on total hip prosthesis. Acta Orthop 2011;82(5):567–76.
21. Kennedy DM, Stratford PW, Hanna SE, et al. Modeling early recovery of physical function following hip and knee arthroplasty. BMC Musculoskelet Disord 2006;7: 100.

22. Davis AM, Perruccio AV, Ibrahim S, et al. The trajectory of recovery and the inter-relationships of symptoms, activity and participation in the first year following total hip and knee replacement. Osteoarthritis Cartilage 2011;19(12):1413–21.

23. Vissers MM, Bussmann JB, Verhaar JA, et al. Recovery of physical functioning after total hip arthroplasty: systematic review and meta-analysis of the literature. Phys Ther 2011;91(5):615–29.

24. Meier W, Mizner RL, Marcus RL, et al. Total knee arthroplasty: muscle impairments, functional limitations, and recommended rehabilitation approaches. J Orthop Sports Phys Ther 2008;38(5):246–56.

25. de Beer J, Petruccelli D, Adili A, et al. Patient perspective survey of total hip vs total knee arthroplasty surgery. J Arthroplasty 2012;27(6):865–9.

26. Bourne RB, Chesworth B, Davis A, et al. Comparing patient outcomes after THA and TKA: IS there a difference? Clin Orthop Relat Res 2010;468(2):542–6.

27. Zhan C, Kaczmarek R, Loyo-Berrios N, et al. Incidence and short-term outcomes of primary and revision hip replacement in the United States. J Bone Joint Surg Am 2007;89(3):526–33.

28. Nguyen-Oghalai TU, Ottenbacher KJ, Caban M, et al. The impact of rheumatoid arthritis on rehabilitation outcomes after lower extremity arthroplasty. J Clin Rheumatol 2007;13(5):247–50.

29. Ito J, Koshino T, Okamoto R, et al. 15-year follow-up study of total knee arthroplasty in patients with rheumatoid arthritis. J Arthroplasty 2003;18(8):984–92.

30. Ethgen O, Bruyere O, Richy F, et al. Health-related quality of life in total hip and total knee arthroplasty. A qualitative and systematic review of the literature. J Bone Joint Surg Am 2004;86–A(5):963–74.

31. Jones CA, Beaupre LA, Johnston DW, et al. Total joint arthroplasties: current concepts of patient outcomes after surgery. Rheum Dis Clin North Am 2007;33(1): 71–86.

32. Jones D, Westby M, Greidanus N, et al. Update on hip and knee arthroplasties: Current state of evidence. Arthritis Rheum 2005;53(5):772–80.

33. McMeeken JM, Galea MP. Impairment of muscle performance before and following total hip replacement. Int J Ther Rehabil 2007;14(2):55–62.

34. McClelland JA, Webster KE, Feller JA. Gait analysis of patients following total knee replacement: a systematic review. Knee 2007;14(4):253–63.

35. Rossi MD, Hasson S. Lower-limb force production in individuals after unilateral total knee arthroplasty. Arch Phys Med Rehabil 2004;85(8):1279–84.

36. Trudelle-Jackson E, Emerson R, Smith S. Outcomes of total hip arthroplasty: a study of patients one year postsurgery. J Orthop Sports Phys Ther 2002;32(6):260–7.

37. Núñez M, Lozano L, Núñez E, et al. Total knee replacement and health-related quality of life: factors influencing long-term outcomes. Arthritis Rheum 2009;61(8): 1062–9.

38. Wylde V, Hewlett S, Learmonth ID, et al. Persistent pain after joint replacement: prevalence, sensory qualities, and postoperative determinants. Pain 2011;152(3): 566–72.

39. Bhave A, Marker DR, Seyler TM, et al. Functional problems and treatment solutions after total hip arthroplasty. J Arthroplasty 2007;22(6 Suppl 2):116–24.

40. Al-Hadithy N, Rozati H, Sewell MD, et al. Causes of a painful total knee arthroplasty. Are patients still receiving total knee arthroplasty for extrinsic pathologies? Int Orthop 2012;36(6):1185–9.

41. Bhave A, Mont M, Tennis S, et al. Functional problems and treatment solutions after total hip and knee joint arthroplasty. J Bone Joint Surg Am 2005;87(Suppl 2):9–21.

42. Brander VA, Stulberg SD, Adams AD, et al. Predicting total knee replacement pain: a prospective, observational study. Clin Orthop Relat Res 2003;416:27–36.

43. Rasch A, Dalén N, Berg HE. Muscle strength, gait, and balance in 20 patients with hip osteoarthritis followed for 2 years after THA. Acta Orthop 2010;81(2):183–8.

44. Shih CH, Du YK, Lin YH, et al. Muscular recovery around the hip joint after total hip arthroplasty. Clin Orthop Relat Res 1994;302:115–20.

45. Mizner RL, Stevens JE, Snyder-Mackler L. Voluntary activation and decreased force production of the quadriceps femoris muscle after total knee arthroplasty. Phys Ther 2003;83(4):359–65.

46. Plaass C, Clauss M, Ochsner PE, et al. Influence of leg length discrepancy on clinical results after total hip arthroplasty–a prospective clinical trial. Hip Int 2011;21(4): 441–9.

47. Swinkels A, Newman JH, Allain TJ. A prospective observational study of falling before and after knee replacement surgery. Age Ageing 2008;38(2):175–81.

48. Milner CE. Is gait normal after total knee arthroplasty? Systematic review of the literature. J Orthop Sci 2009;14:114–20.

49. Walsh M, Woodhouse LJ, Thomas SG, et al. Physical impairments and functional limitations: a comparison of individuals 1 year after total knee arthroplasty with control subjects. Phys Ther 1998;78(3):248–58.

50. Noble PC, Gordon MJ, Weiss JM, et al. Does total knee replacement restore normal knee function? Orthop Relat Res 2005(431):157–65.

51. Franklin PD, Li W, Ayers DC. Functional outcome after total knee replacement varies with patient attributes. Clin Orthop Relat Res 2008;466:2597–604.

52. Bade MJ, Stevens-Lapsley JE. Restoration of physical function in patients following total knee arthroplasty: an update on rehabilitation practices. Curr Opin Rheumatol 2012;24(2):208–14.

53. Jones DL. A public health perspective on physical activity after total hip or knee arthroplasty for osteoarthritis. Physician Sportsmed 2011;39(4):70–9.

54. Hootman JM, Macera CA, Ham SA, et al. Physical activity levels among the general US adult population and in adults with and without arthritis. Arthritis Rheum 2003; 49(1):129–35.

55. Wagenmakers R, Stevens M, Zijlstra W, et al. Habitual physical activity behavior of patients after primary total hip arthroplasty. Phys Ther 2008;88(9):1039–48.

56. Hayes DA, Watts MC, Anderson LJ, et al. Knee arthroplasty: a cross-sectional study assessing energy expenditure and activity. ANZ J Surg 2010;81:371–4.

57. Williams DH, Greidanus NV, Masri BA, et al. Predictors of participation in sports after hip and knee arthroplasty. Clin Orthop Relat Res 2012;470:555–61.

58. Naal FD, Impellizzeri FM. How active are patients undergoing total joint arthroplasty? A systematic review. Clin Orthop Relat Res 2010;468(7):1891–904.

59. Waciakowski D, Urban K. Comparative outcomes of total knee arthroplasty on physically active and passive patients. Acta Medica 2011;54(2):69–72.

60. Rastogi R, Davis AM, Chesworth BM. A cross-sectional look at patient concerns in the first six weeks following primary total knee arthroplasty. Health Qual Life Outcomes 2007;5:48. Available at: http://www.hqlo.com/content/5/1/48. Accessed May 3, 2012.

61. Wylde V, Dieppe P, Hewlett S, et al. Total knee replacement: is it really an effective procedure for all? Knee 2007;14(6):417–23.

62. Kauppila AM, Kyllönen E, Ohtonen P, et al. Outcomes of primary total knee arthroplasty: the impact of patient-relevant factors on self-reported function and quality of life. Disabil Rehabil 2011;33(17-18):1659–67.

63. Higuera Ca, Elsharkawy K, Klika AK, et al. Predictors of early adverse outcomes after knee and hip arthroplasty in geriatric patients. Clin Orthop Relat Res 2011;469(5): 1391–400.
64. Clement ND, MacDonald D, Howie CR, et al. The outcome of primary total hip and knee arthroplasty in patients aged 80 years or more. J Bone Joint Surg Br 2011;93–B(9):1265–70.
65. Loeser RF. Age-related changes in the musculoskeletal system and the development of osteoarthritis. Clin Geriatr Med 2010;26(3):371–86.
66. Evered LA, Silbert BS, Scott DA, et al. Preexisting cognitive impairment and mild cognitive impairment in subjects presenting for total hip joint replacement. Anesthesiology 2011;114(6):1297–304.
67. Stroh DA, Delanois R, Naziri O, et al. Total knee arthroplasty in patients over 80 years of age. J Knee Surg 2011;24(4):279–83.
68. Hamel MB, Toth M, Legedza A, et al. Joint replacement surgery in elderly patients with severe osteoarthritis of the hip or knee: decision making, postoperative recovery, and clinical outcomes. Arch Intern Med 2008;168(13):1430–40.
69. Carli F, Zavorsky GS. Optimizing functional exercise capacity in the elderly surgical population. Curr Opin Nutr Metab Care 2005;8:23–32.
70. Clark BC, Manini TM. Functional consequences of sarcopenia and dynapenia in the elderly. Curr Opin Nutr Metab Care 2010;13:271–6.
71. Cipriano LE, Chesworth BM, Anderson CK, et al. Predicting joint replacement waiting times. Health Care Manag Sci 2007;10(2):195–215.
72. Canadian Institute of Health Information. Wait times in Canada—a comparison by province, 2011. Healthc Q 2011;14(2):108. Available at: secure.cihi.ca/cihiweb/products/Wait_times_tables_2011_en.pdf. Accessed January 15, 2012.
73. Coyte PC, Wright JG, Hawker GA, et al. Waiting times for knee-replacement surgery in the United States and Ontario. N Engl J Med 1994;331(16):1068–71.
74. Ackerman IN, Bennell KL, Osborne RH. Decline in health-related quality of life reported by more than half of those waiting for joint replacement surgery: a prospective cohort study. BMC Musculoskelet Disord 2011;12:108. Available at: http://www.biomedcentral.com/1471-2474/12/108. Accessed December 12, 2011.
75. Hoogeboom TJ, van den Ende CH, van der Sluis G, et al. The impact of waiting for total joint replacement on pain and functional status: a systematic review. Osteoarthritis Cartilage 2009;17(11):1420–7.
76. Lucas B. Preparing patients for hip and knee replacement surgery. Nurs Standard 2007;22(2):50–6.
77. Philbin EF, Groff GD, Ries MD, et al. Cardiovascular fitness and health in patients with end-stage osteoarthritis. Arthritis Rheum 1995;38(6):799–805.
78. McDonald S, Hetrick S, Green S. Pre-operative education for hip or knee replacement. Cochrane Database Syst Rev 2004;1:CD003526.
79. Ackerman IL, Bennell KL. Does pre-operative physiotherapy improve outcomes from lower limb joint replacement surgery? A systematic review. Aust J Physiother 2004;50(1):25–30.
80. Coudeyre E, Jardin C, Givron P, et al. Could preoperative rehabilitation modify postoperative outcomes after total hip and knee arthroplasty? Elaboration of French clinical practice guidelines. Ann Readapt Med Phys 2007;50(3):189–97.
81. Rooks DS, Huang J, Bierbarum BE, et al. Effect of preoperative exercise on measures of functional status in men and women undergoing total hip and knee arthroplasty. Arthritis Rheum (Arthritis Care Res) 2006;55(5):700–8.

82. Topp R, Swank AM, Quesada PM, et al. The effect of prehabilitation exercise on strength and functioning after total knee arthroplasty. Phys Med Rehabil 2009;1(8): 729–35.
83. Swank AM, Kachelman JB, Bibeau W, et al. Prehabilitation before total knee arthroplasty increases strength and function in older adults with severe osteoarthritis. J Strength Cond Res 2011;25(2):318–25.
84. Daltroy LH, Morlino CI, Eaton HM, et al. Preoperative education for total hip and knee replacement patients. Arthritis Care Res 1998;11(6):469–78.
85. Ayers DC, Franklin PD, Trief PM, et al. Psychological attributes of preoperative total joint replacement patients: implications for optimal physical outcomes. J Arthroplasty 2004;19(7 Suppl 2):125–30.
86. Barbieri A, Vanhaecht K, Van Herck P, et al. Effects of clinical pathways in the joint replacement: a meta-analysis. BMC Med 2009;7:32. Available at: http://www.biomedcentral.com/1741-7015/7/32. Accessed October 11, 2011.
87. Bukowski E. Practice guideline: acute care management following total hip arthroplasty (postoperative days 1-4). Orthop Phys Ther Pract 2005;17(3):10–4.
88. Bizzini M, Boldt J, Munzinger U, et al. Rehabilitation guidelines after total knee arthroplasty. Orthopade 2003;32(6):527–34.
89. Enloe LJ, Shields RK, Smith K, et al. Total hip and knee replacement treatment programs: a report using consensus. J Orthop Sports Phys Ther 1996;23(1):3–11.
90. Khan F, Ng L, Gonzalez S, et al. Multidisciplinary rehabilitation programmes following joint replacement at the hip and knee in chronic arthropathy. Cochrane Database Syst Rev 2008;2:CD004957.
91. Minns Lowe CJ, Barker KL, Dewey ME, et al. Effectiveness of physiotherapy exercise following hip arthroplasty for osteoarthritis: a systematic review of clinical trials. BMC Musculoskelet Disord 2009;10:98.
92. Minns Lowe CJ, Barker KL, Dewey M, et al. Effectiveness of physiotherapy exercise after knee arthroplasty for osteoarthritis: systematic review and meta-analysis of randomised controlled trials. Br Med J 2007;335(7624):812.
93. Di Monaco M, Vallero F, Tappero R, et al. Rehabilitation after total hip arthroplasty: a systematic review of controlled trials on physical exercise programs. Eur J Phys Rehabil Med 2009;45:303–17.
94. Okoro T, Lemmey AB, Maddison P, et al. An appraisal of rehabilitation regimes used for improving functional outcome after total hip replacement surgery. Sports Med Arthrosc Rehabil Ther Technol. 2012;4:5. Available at: http://www.smarttjournal.com/content/4/1/5. Accessed February 9, 2012.
95. Petterson SC, Mizner RL, Stevens JE, et al. Improved function from progressive strengthening interventions after total knee arthroplasty: a randomized clinical trial with an imbedded prospective cohort. Arthritis Rheum 2009;61(2):174–83.
96. Harmer AR, Naylor JM, Crosbie J, et al. Land-based versus water-based rehabilitation following total knee replacement: a randomized, single-blind trial. Arthritis Rheum 2009;61(2):184–91.
97. Coulter CL, Weber JM, Scarvell JM. Group physiotherapy provides similar outcomes for participants after joint replacement surgery as 1-to-1 physiotherapy: a sequential cohort study. Arch Phys Med Rehabil 2009;90(10):1727–33.
98. Kramer JF, Speechley M, Bourne R, et al. Comparison of clinic- and home-based rehabilitation programs after total knee arthroplasty. Clin Orthop 2003(410):225–34.
99. Scherak O, Kolarz G, Wottawa A, et al. Comparison between early and late inpatient rehabilitation measures after implantation of total hip endoprostheses. Rehabilitation 1998;37(3):123–7.

100. Trudelle-Jackson E, Smith SS. Effects of a late-phase exercise program after total hip arthroplasty: a randomized controlled trial. Arch Phys Med Rehabil 2004;85(7): 1056–62.

101. Jan MH, Hung JY, Lin JC, et al. Effects of a home program on strength, walking speed, and function after total hip replacement. Arch Phys Med Rehabil 2004; 85(12):1943–51.

102. LaStayo PC, Meier W, Marcus RL, et al. Reversing muscle and mobility deficits 1 to 4 years after TKA: a pilot study. Clin Orthop Relat Res 2009;467(6):1493–500.

103. Liebs TR, Herzberg W, Rüther W, et al. Multicenter randomized controlled trial comparing early versus late aquatic therapy after total hip or knee arthroplasty. Arch Phys Med Rehabil 2012;93(2):192–9.

104. Naylor JM, Mittal R, Carroll K, et al. Introductory insights into patient preferences for outpatient rehabilitation after knee replacement: implications for practice and future research. J Eval Clin Pract 2012;18(3):586–92.

105. Garber CE, Blissmer B, Deschenes MR, et al. American College of Sports Medicine position stand. Quantity and quality of exercise for developing and maintaining cardiorespiratory, musculoskeletal, and neuromotor fitness in apparently healthy adults: guidance for prescribing exercise. Med Sci Sports Exerc 2011;43(7): 1334–59.

106. American College of Sports Medicine. American College of Sports Medicine position stand. Progression models in resistance training for healthy adults. Med Sci Sports Exerc 2009;41(3):687–708.

107. Ulrich SD, Bhave A, Marker DR, et al. Focused rehabilitation treatment of poorly functioning total knee arthroplasties. Clin Orthop Relat Res 2007;464:138–45.

108. Foley A, Hillier S, Barnard R. Effectiveness of once-weekly gym-based exercise programmes for older adults post discharge from day rehabilitation: a randomised controlled trial. Br J Sports Med 2011;45:978–86.

109. World Health Organization. International classification of functioning, disability and health (ICF). Published 2001. Available at: http://www.who.int/classifications/icf/. Accessed March 3, 2004.

110. Lopez-Olivo MA, Landon GC, Siff SJ, et al. Psychosocial determinants of outcomes in knee replacement. Ann Rheum Dis 2011;70(10):1775–81.

111. Baumann C, Rat AC, Osnowycz G, et al. Do clinical presentation and pre-operative quality of life predict satisfaction with care after total hip or knee replacement? J Bone Joint Surg Br 2006;88(3):366–73.

112. Bourne RB, McCalden RW, MacDonald SJ, et al. Influence of patient factors on TKA outcomes at 5 to 11 years followup. Clin Orthop 2007(464):27–31.

113. Brander VA, Gondek S, Martin E, et al. Pain and depression influence outcome 5 years after knee replacement surgery. Clin Orthop Relat Res 2007;464:21–6.

114. Brander VA, Malhotra S, Jet J, et al. Outcome of hip and knee arthroplasty in persons aged 80 years and older. Clin Orthop Relat Res 1997(345):67–78.

115. Farin E, Glattacker M, Jackel WH. Predictors of rehabilitation outcome in patients after total hip and total knee arthroplasty–a multilevel analysis. Physikalische Medizin Rehabilitationsmedizin Kurortmedizin 2006;16(2):82–91.

116. Mahomed NN, Liang MH, Cook EF, et al. The importance of patient expectations in predicting functional outcomes after total joint arthroplasty. J Rheumatol 2002;29(6): 1273–9.

117. Naylor JM, Harmer AR, Heard RC. Severe other joint disease and obesity independently influence recovery after joint replacement surgery: an observational study. Aust J Physiother 2008;54(1):57–64.

118. van den Akker-Scheek I, Stevens M, Groothoff JW, et al. Preoperative or postoperative self-efficacy: which is a better predictor of outcome after total hip or knee arthroplasty? Patient Educ Couns 2007;66(1):92–9.

119. Young NL, Cheah D, Waddell JP, et al. Patient characteristics that affect the outcome of total hip arthroplasty: a review. Can J Surg 1998;41(3):188–95.

120. Baumann C, Rat AC, Mainard D, et al. Importance of patient satisfaction with care in predicting osteoarthritis-specific health-related quality of life one year after total joint arthroplasty. Qual Life Res 2011;20(10):1581–8.

121. Vissers MM, Bussmann JB, Verhaar JA, et al. Psychological factors affecting the outcome of total hip and knee arthroplasty: a systematic review. Semin Arthritis Rheum 2012;41(4):576–88.

122. Bischoff-Ferrari HA, Lingard EA, Baron JA, et al. Psychosocial and geriatric correlates of functional status after total hip replacement. Arthritis Care Res 2004;51(5):829–35.

123. Sullivan M, Tanzer M, Reardon G, et al. The role of presurgical expectancies in predicting pain and function one year following total knee arthroplasty. Pain 2011;152:2287–93.

124. Shervin N, Rubash HE, Katz JN. Orthopaedic procedure volume and patient outcomes: a systematic literature review. Clin Orthop Relat Res 2007;457:35–41.

Physical Activity Participation Among Patients After Total Hip and Knee Arthroplasty

Martin Stevens, PhD[a],*, Inge H.F. Reininga, PhD[b,c],
Sjoerd K. Bulstra, MD, PhD[a], Robert Wagenmakers, MD, PhD[d],
Inge van den Akker-Scheek, PhD[a]

KEYWORDS

- Older adults • Osteoarthritis • Physical activity • Total hip arthroplasty
- Total knee arthroplasty

KEY POINTS

- For older adults there are important beneficial effects of regular physical activity after total hip arthroplasty (THA)/total knee arthroplasty (TKA), not only from a general health perspective but also specifically after THA/TKA.
- Approximately half of post THA/TKA patients do not meet the health-enhancing physical activity guidelines; it is especially important for patients after THA/TKA to remain or become physically active.

INTRODUCTION

In Western society, regular physical activity is considered to be one of the most important lifestyle behaviors affecting health.[1] Regular physical activity has been shown to be effective in primary and secondary prevention of several chronic health conditions and is linked with a reduction in all-cause mortality.[1–3] It also enhances musculoskeletal fitness.

Musculoskeletal fitness refers to muscular strength, muscular endurance, and joint flexibility. Musculoskeletal fitness is positively associated with functional autonomy in

DISCLOSURE: All authors disclose that they do not have any relationship with a commercial company that has a direct financial interest in the subject discussed in the article.

[a] Department of Orthopedics, University of Groningen, University Medical Center, P.O. Box 30001, Hanzeplein 1, 9700 RB Groningen, The Netherlands; [b] Department of Traumatology, University of Groningen, University Medical Center, Hanzeplein 1, 9700 RB Groningen, The Netherlands; [c] Department of Orthopedics, Martini Hospital, Van Swietenplein 1, 9728 NT Groningen, The Netherlands; [d] Department of Orthopedics, Amphia Hospital, Langendijk 75, 4819 EV Breda, The Netherlands
* Corresponding author.
E-mail address: m.stevens@umcg.nl

older adults.[4] At the same time, a lack of physical activity is considered a potential burden on public health, and is associated with premature death as a result of coronary heart disease, colon cancer, and non–insulin-dependent diabetes.[1] Current recommendations for health-enhancing physical activity are based on the guidelines of the American College of Sports Medicine and the American Heart Association, published in 2007.[2,3] These guidelines recommend that every healthy adult aged 18 to 65 perform moderate-intensity aerobic (endurance) physical activity for 30 minutes or more at least 5 days per week, or vigorous-intensity aerobic physical activity for a minimum of 20 minutes at least 3 days per week.

Osteoarthritis (OA) is among the most prevalent age-related musculoskeletal conditions. Although OA may affect any joint of the body, it is most commonly seen in the hip and knee.[5] OA of the hip or knee leads to significant impairment in patients' ability to perform activities of daily living and has a great impact on health-related quality of life.[6,7] In advanced OA of the hip or knee, total hip and knee arthroplasty (THA/TKA) are highly successful and widely applied operative treatments, with 208,600 primary THAs and 450,000 TKAs performed in the United States in 2005[8] and 20,451 THAs and 20,266 TKAs in The Netherlands in 2008.[9] Because of growth of the older population and changing thresholds for surgery, these numbers are expected to increase dramatically in the coming decades.[8,9]

Although THA and TKA are highly successful, little is known about the physical activity behavior of patients after THA/TKA. The scarce knowledge we have is mainly limited to its role as an important negative determinant of prosthetic wear and loosening, affecting the longevity of the total hip or knee prosthesis.[10–12] However, for older adults there are important beneficial effects of regular physical activity after THA/TKA, not only from a general health perspective, but also in that it specifically benefits the prosthesis. The objective of this paper is to review (1) the benefits of physical activity for patients after THA/TKA, (2) the potential negative consequences of physical activity on hip or knee prosthesis, (3) the measurement of physical activity, (4) physical activity behavior, and (5) the current opinion of health care professionals regarding types of physical activities recommended for patients after THA/TKA.

ADVANTAGES AND CONSIDERATIONS OF PHYSICAL ACTIVITY

Regular physical activity has several general health benefits, the prevention of chronic conditions, including cardiovascular disease, type 2 diabetes, colon and breast cancers, hypertension, obesity, depression, and osteoporosis, and is linked to a reduction in all-cause mortality.[1,13–15] For older people, like most total joint arthroplasty patients, regular physical activity can delay the age-related decline in musculoskeletal fitness. Musculoskeletal fitness is positively associated with functional autonomy, mobility, and bone health, and negatively associated with the risks of falls.[13,14] A certain level of musculoskeletal fitness is needed to live independently, which is a valued component of overall quality of life for older persons.[16]

Being regularly physically active enhances muscle strength, balance, and coordination, which has proven to prevent falls.[17,18] Each year, about 30% of community-dwelling older adults fall. As a result, approximately 5% sustain fractures and an additional 5% to 11% sustain other serious injuries.[19] For those with a joint prosthesis, these falls can result in periprosthetic fracture, implant loosening, and/or dislocation of a hip prosthesis, and may cause serious morbidity.

There are indications that increased bone density owing to physical activity improves fixation of the prosthesis, reducing the risk of prosthetic loosening.[20–22] Physical activity might also minimize bone loss owing to stress shielding.[23] Stress shielding refers to the reduction of bone density as a result of removal of normal stress from the bone by an implant. Moreover, because preservation of the quality and quantity of cortical bone is important, should revision become necessary, this facilitates any future revision surgery.

There are some negative consequences for patients after total joint arthroplasty. One of the most important consequences of physical activity is wear of the prosthesis; it results in polyethylene particles and subsequently in prosthetic loosening. This may limit the longevity of the implant. Although it is said that the longevity of a total joint prosthesis is 15 to 20 years, prosthesis wear is considered to be a function of use, not of time in situ.[10] The degree of prosthesis wear, however, is not solely related to physical activity. Patient- and prosthesis-related factors also contribute to the longevity of the prosthesis.[11] Moreover, the degree of prosthesis wear depends not only on the number of steps, but also on the mechanical loading of the joint. The amount of this loading, in turn, depends on body weight and type of physical activity. Kuster[24] reported the load on the hip and knee joint of several types of physical activities. In general, it can be concluded that activities with high-peak loading, like running, cause more mechanical loading of the joint than physical activities like walking and cycling, and may cause more wear of the prosthesis. Because mechanical loading of the joint also depends on the amount of body weight of the patient (patient-related factor), the load on the joint is higher during each activity for patients with a higher body weight. Overweight (body mass index [BMI] 25–30 kg/m^2) and obesity (BMI >30 kg/m^2) negatively affect prosthetic longevity as well as the general health of patients. Studies have found a correlation between obesity and the risk of aseptic loosening of the prosthesis.[12,25] Although obese patients often claim that the OA in their joint(s) limits their ability to perform physical activities, studies have shown that THA or TKA does not typically lead to weight loss.[26,27] A higher BMI has even been shown to be associated with lower physical activity in patients after THA.[28] For these reasons, physical activity programs are needed for overweight and obese patients after total joint arthroplasty to increase energy expenditure and lower their body weight.

PHYSICAL ACTIVITY MEASURES

Physical activity behavior is challenging to measure for a number of reasons. Instruments need to be valid and reproducible, and provide a detailed profile of type, duration, frequency, and intensity of the most common daily physical activities of patients after THA/TKA. They should not be too expensive when used for large-scale studies and should be able to assess physical activity at the individual as well as at the group levels. Moreover, they should not interfere with the performed physical activity, and need to be acceptable to the patient and applicable to different age groups.[1,29] They should also account for the variations in physical activity that may occur over time. For this reason, the activity score should be cumulative and assessed on a regular basis.[29] Unfortunately, none of the instruments in use today that measure physical activity fulfills all of these criteria.

Physical activity can be assessed by direct measurements, including behavioral observation; mechanical or electronic devices, such as heart rate monitors, pedometers, motion sensors, or accelerometers; physiologic measurements such as direct and indirect calorimetry; or by self-report, including diaries, logs, recall surveys, retrospective quantitative histories, and global self-reports.[1]

Until now, self-report measures have been the most widely used type of physical activity measure, allowing collection of data from different domains of physical activity from a large number of people at low costs. There are limitations, however, to their use. Recalling physical activity is a highly complex cognitive task and instruments may vary in their cognitive demands. Older adults in particular may have memory and recall skill limitations. Another problem is that people tend to overestimate their physical activity level.[30] Because of the limitation of self-report measures, there is an increasing tendency to use pedometers and accelerometers as direct ways of measurement. Until now their use was limited owing to high costs and the burden on participants and investigators. Furthermore, they frequently provide only information about certain aspects of physical functioning or movement and typically can only be used in a limited time frame. A major advantage of direct measurements, however, is that they eliminate the problems of poor memory and biased self-reporting, and thus can be considered an objective method for assessing physical activity.

Self-Report Instruments: Measures of Ability to Participate in Physical Activities

There are different measures, mainly physician-based and self-reported disease-specific and generic measures, that have been used for outcome assessment after THA/TKA, such as the Harris Hip Score,[31] the Knee Society Score,[32] the Oxford Hip and Knee Scores,[33] the Knee Injury and Osteoarthritis Outcome Score,[34] the Hip disability and Osteoarthritis Outcome Score,[35] the Western Ontario and McMaster Universities Osteoarthritis Index,[36] and the MOS 36-Item Short Form Health Survey.[37] It has been shown, however, that outcome measures like the Western Ontario and McMaster Universities Osteoarthritis Index or Harris Hip Score, which measure physical functioning, are clinically not useful to predict the physical activity *behavior* of patients after THA.[38] This result is in line with a study into the predictive power of the Harris Hip Score on activity level.[39] It probably reflects the fact that, with respect to physical functioning, these outcome measures only assess functional limitations, whereas physical activity behavior is determined by many other factors, including demographic, social, psychological, and environmental dynamics.[40] It can be concluded that the ability to participate in physical activities or functional limitations and physical activity behavior are 2 different aspects of physical functioning, and should therefore be assessed with different measures.

Self-Report Instruments: Measures of Physical Activity Behaviors

Presently, the UCLA activity score[41] and the Grimby scale[42] are commonly used in orthopedics to categorize patients according to their physical activity level. These scoring tools categorize the activity level of patients, but fail to provide detailed information on duration, frequency and energy expenditure of patients' activities and consequently provide no estimation of metabolic equivalent of task, which makes comparing scores across measures difficult. Furthermore, it does not allow assessment of compliance with the recommendations for health-enhancing physical activity. To our knowledge neither scoring instrument has been validated until recently.

Other self-report instruments that might be better suited to measuring physical activity are the International Physical Assessment Questionnaire (IPAQ)[43] and the Short Questionnaire to Assess Physical Activity (SQUASH).[44] Although the IPAQ and the SQUASH are hampered by some of the mentioned limitations with self-report instruments, both are short, easy to complete, and address several domains of habitual physical activity. The recall period of physical activities is during an average week in the past months. To overcome the problem of multiple physical activity questionnaires, the IPAQ was developed as an instrument for cross-national monitoring of physical activity and inactivity.[30] Although it has not been validated for post-THA and -TKA patients, it can be presumed that the IPAQ can be useful for assessing their overall physical activity levels (even though, as an epidemiologic instrument, the IPAQ was not developed for use in clinical settings in the first place or for measuring change as a function of physical activity interventions). The SQUASH is used nationwide in The Netherlands. Government agencies use it to monitor the physical activity level of the Dutch population. The reliability and validity of this questionnaire have been specifically determined in a population of patients after THA.[45] To date, no gold standard for the assessment of physical activity has been determined and there is no physical activity questionnaire that has been validated for both TKA and THA patients.

Objective Instruments: Accelerometry

Although self-reported physical activity questionnaires are the most frequently employed assessment tool at a population level, novel body-fixed sensor-based technology, such as accelerometers, can provide an objective insight into habitual physical activity of patients after THA/TKA. Accelerometers are mostly worn on the waist and measure and record time-varying accelerations of the body. The summation of accelerations measured during a user-specified time interval (epoch) are collected and reported in "counts." These counts represent the intensity of activity in that epoch. In this way frequency, duration, total volume, and intensity of physical activity can be assessed. New generations of accelerometers use sophisticated data-processing approaches, allowing pattern recognition of physical activity.[46] This allows for detailed profiling not only of physical activity, but also of inactivity.[46] In this way, a more comprehensive exploration of the links between health and frequency, intensity, and duration of physical activity will become possible.[46] Objective assessment of physical functioning can also be used to evaluate the result of orthopedic procedures such as THA/TKA.[39] However, to obtain clear insight into physical activity behavior, it is advised to use both self-reported and objective instruments.

MEASURING SEDENTARY BEHAVIOR

Besides the focus on physical activity behavior, there is increasing attention on time spent on sedentary activities, such as prolonged TV watching. Research has indicated that sedentary behavior, measured as TV viewing time or overall sitting time, reduces a person's life expectancy and is linked with an increased risk for overweight, type 2 diabetes, cardiometabolic risk, and the metabolic syndrome, which could not (totally) be explained by reduced amount of physical activity and an unhealthy diet that is often associated with sitting and watching TV.[47–50] This indicates that sedentary behavior itself has to be considered a risk factor. Sedentary behavior is often determined by self-report questionnaires, asking to report sitting time or television viewing time. Objectively, sedentary behavior can be determined with the use of accelerometry.[51] To date, no research is performed yet on the sedentary behavior of patients after THA/TKA.

PHYSICAL ACTIVITY AFTER THA AND TKA
Total Hip Arthroplasty

So far, limited research is available about physical activity behavior after THA and TKA. For THA patients, both a retrospective and a prospective cohort study were conducted at our institute. In a retrospective study, 273 patients participated who had undergone a primary THA (minimum of 1 year postoperatively).[52] Physical activity was measured with the SQUASH questionnaire. Comparisons were made with a normative population consisting of inhabitants from the same geographical region as the study population. The mean age of the respondents was 62.7 (SD 13.7) years and mostly female (60.8%). The patients spent in total 1601 (SD 1327) minutes per week on physical activity and 51.2% met the recommendation of health-enhancing physical activity, compared with 48.8% in the normative population. Most of the physical activity time was spent doing household and leisure activities. No differences were found between the patients and the normative group with respect to amount of physical activity and meeting the recommendation. Patients with THA tended to spend more time in activities of light and moderate intensity and less time in activities of vigorous intensity compared with the normative group.

In a prospective study of 653 participants the SQUASH was used.[53] The mean age of respondents was 70.3 (SD 8.2) years and mostly female (74.0%). Participants were physically active a mean of 1468 (SD 1138) minutes per week. Most time was spent in household and leisure activities. Younger participants (≤75 years) were physically more active than older participants. A lower BMI was predictive of a higher level of physical activity. Sixty-seven percent of the participants adhered to the guidelines of health-enhancing physical activity. The guidelines were met more often by younger participants, male participants, and those without problems in the lower extremities. The results of this prospective study (at 1 year postoperatively) reveal a slightly lower total amount of physical activity than the retrospective study (1–5 years postoperatively), perhaps because the mean age of the patients was lower. It also might reflect a slight further increase of physical activity in the years after the surgery. As in the prospective study, most of the time was spent in household activities and leisure time activities, and mostly light-intensity activities were performed. Comparison of the results of both studies with those of previous studies is hampered by the fact that level of physical activity has been determined predominantly by means of categorical scoring tools such as the UCLA Activity Score[41] and the Grimby scale.[42] However, results of studies that used the UCLA Activity Score indicate a moderate activity level in patients at least 3 years after THA.[54–56] Using the Grimby scale, a light- to moderate-intensity activity level was found in patients 1 to 2 years after THA.[57] When interpreting these results, it should be noted that these studies differ from ours not only with respect to the scoring tool used, but also the populations in which physical activity was measured and the point of follow-up. It can be nonetheless concluded that their results are more or less in line with our research, where mostly light-intensity activities followed by moderate-intensity activities were undertaken by the patients.

Total Knee Arthroplasty

Previous studies on physical activity after TKA concentrate mainly on a return to sports activities.[58–60] A retrospective cohort study was conducted at our institute with 844 participants. Habitual physical activity behavior and the extent to which they adhered to international guidelines for health-enhancing physical activity were measured 1 to 5 years postoperatively. Before enrollment, time after surgery was at least 1 year. The mean age of respondents was 72.0 years (SD 9.3) and most were female (74.1%). Physical activity was measured with the SQUASH questionnaire. Data from these patients were compared with a normative population consisting of inhabitants from the same geographical region as the study population. The TKA patients spent a total of 1347 (SD 1278) minutes per week on physical activity, mostly of light intensity (780 [SD 874] min/wk), and in the household and leisure time activity categories. Patients younger than 65 years spent significantly more time on physical activity than patients older than 65 years. Although there was no difference in total amount of physical activity between male and female patients, there were significant differences between males and females with intensity of activity. Female TKA patients spent significantly more time on light-intensity activities, whereas a significant difference in favor of male patients was seen for moderate- and high-intensity activities. Compared with the normative group, TKA patients spent significantly less time on the total amount of physical activity per week and met the guidelines for health-enhancing physical activity less often (55% vs 64%). The total amount of physical activity were congruent with that of the results reported by Brandes and colleagues,[61] who also concluded that TKA patients are less active than healthy counterparts, although they only measured until 1 year postoperatively. Male gender and age younger than 65 years increased the chances of meeting the physical activity guidelines.

Overall, it can be concluded that information of physical activity behavior of patients after THA and TKA remains scarce. Information available indicates that patients are less active or as active compared with people in the general population. This encompasses that approximately half of patients do not meet the health enhancing physical activity guidelines; it is especially important for patients after THA/TKA to remain or become physically active. However, more research is needed to draw definite conclusions about the physical activity behavior of patients after THA/TKA.

RECOMMENDATIONS

To date, there are limited data to guide orthopedic surgeons' recommendations regarding leisure time and sports activities after THA/TKA. Current recommendations of health-enhancing physical activity are based on the position stands of the American College of Sports Medicine and the American Heart Association, which were published in 2007.[2,3] As mentioned, these guidelines recommend that every healthy adult aged 18 to 65 years perform moderate-intensity aerobic (endurance) physical activity for 30 minutes or more at least 5 days per week, or vigorous-intensity aerobic physical activity for a minimum of 20 minutes at least 3 days per week. In general, these recommendations also apply to older adults (age ≥65 years). In a survey conducted at our institute, Dutch orthopedic surgeons were asked if they were aware of the existence of health-enhancing physical activity recommendations. Forty percent of the surgeons answered positively, and about one third (34%) also reported that they advise THA/TKA patients to comply with these recommendations.

The recommendations for health-enhancing physical activity provide information about frequency, intensity, and duration of physical activities, but not about type of physical activities. Type of physical activity is particularly important for patients after THA/TKA, because mechanical loading applied to the prosthesis differs between different physical activities and may influence prosthetic wear and subsequent loosening. Furthermore, certain physical activities, such as contact sports, may increase the risk of falls, thereby posing a risk factor for sustaining a dislocation of a hip prosthesis or a periprosthetic fracture. Available recommendations about type of activity are mainly based on research done in American studies[62-66] that evaluated orthopedic surgeons' preferences, leading to consensus guidelines. However, leisure time and sports activities are, to a certain extent, culturally based. We therefore conducted a study assessing the current standards of the Dutch orthopedic community for recommendations for physical activity after THA/TKA. In general, for THA as well as TKA patients, low- and moderate-impact activities (such as walking, bicycling, and yoga/tai-chi) were allowed or allowed if patients had previous experience with these activities.[67] Contact sports were not allowed (**Table 1**). It can be concluded that the recommendations of Dutch orthopedic surgeons on physical activities after THA are more or less in line with those of their American colleagues,[62-64,66] who do not recommend contact sports or high-impact activities either. Dutch orthopedic surgeons tended to be slightly more conservative in allowing certain physical activities. The recommendations are also in line with recent a report from Germany.[68]

Table 1
Advice after a total hip or knee arthroplasty

Leisure Time or Sports Activity	Advice with a Total Hip Arthroplasty		Advice with a Total Knee Arthroplasty	
	<65 Years	>65 Years	<65 Years	>65 Years
Aerobics	Allow with experience	Allow with experience	Allow with experience	Allow with experience
Water aerobics	Allow	Allow	Allow	Allow
Badminton	Undecided	Undecided	Undecided	Undecided
Basketball	Not allowed	Not allowed	Not allowed	Not allowed
Dancing	Allow	Allow	Allow	Allow
Bicycling	Allow	Allow	Allow	Allow
Fitness	Allow	Allow	Allow	Allow
Martial arts	Not allowed	Not allowed	Not allowed	Not allowed
Golf	Allow	Allow	Allow	Allow
Gymnastics	Undecided	Undecided	Undecided	Undecided
Handball	Not allowed	Not allowed	Not allowed	Not allowed
Jogging	Undecided	Undecided	Not allowed	Not allowed
Treadmill running	Undecided	Undecided	Undecided	Undecided
Field hockey	Undecided	Not allowed	Not allowed	Not allowed
Jeu de boules/boule	Allow	Allow	Allow	Allow
Canoeing	Allow with experience	Allow with experience	Allow with experience	Allow with experience
Korfball	Not allowed	Not allowed	Not allowed	Not allowed
Cross-country skiing	Allow with experience	Allow with experience	Allow with experience	Allow with experience
Nordic walking	Allow	Allow	Allow	Allow
Horseback riding	Allow with experience	Allow with experience	Allow with experience	Allow with experience
Rowing	Allow with experience	Allow with experience	Allow	Allow with experience
Ice skating	Allow with experience	Allow with experience	Allow with experience	Allow with experience
Skiing	Allow with experience	Undecided	Undecided	Undecided
Snowboarding	Undecided	Not allowed	Not allowed	Not allowed
Squash	Undecided	Undecided	Undecided	Undecided
Surfing	Undecided	Undecided	Allow with experience	Undecided
Table tennis	Allow with experience	Allow with experience	Allow with experience	Allow with experience
Singles tennis	Allow with experience	Undecided	Undecided	Undecided
Doubles tennis	Allow with experience	Allow with experience	Allow with experience	Allow with experience
Field soccer	Not allowed	Not allowed	Not allowed	Not allowed
Indoor soccer	Not allowed	Not allowed	Not allowed	Not allowed

(continued on next page)

Table 1 (continued)				
	Advice with a Total Hip Arthroplasty		**Advice with a Total Knee Arthroplasty**	
Leisure Time or Sports Activity	**<65 Years**	**>65 Years**	**<65 Years**	**>65 Years**
Volleyball	Undecided	Not allowed	Not allowed	Not allowed
Walking	Allow	Allow	Allow	Allow
Road cycling	Allow with experience	Allow with experience	Allow with experience	Allow with experience
Yoga/tai chi	Allow with experience	Allow with experience	Allow with experience	Allow with experience
Sailing	Allow with experience	Allow with experience	Allow with experience	Allow with experience
Swimming	Allow	Allow	Allow	Allow

With respect to TKA, the Dutch research can be compared with that of McGrory and associates,[62] Healy and colleagues,[65] and Swanson and co-workers,[63] although the latter only looked at a selected number of physical activities. For example, contact sports were not included. In general, Swanson and colleagues[63] and Healy and associates[65] allowed low-impact but not high-impact activities. McGrory and colleagues[62] included contact sports and came to the same conclusion we did. In Europe, Kuster[24] published a review of the literature, and the conclusions are in line with ours.

One must keep in mind that both American and Dutch recommendations for physical activity after THA/TKA are based on consensus among orthopedic surgeons. In that sense, there is no real scientific evidence for the guidelines. Hence, future research is needed that focuses on the connection between different leisure time and sports activities and prosthetic wear. Finally, it must be emphasized that the results of these studies can only serve as parameters. When advising a patient on returning to leisure time or sports activities after THA/TKA, these guidelines must be tailored to the personal circumstances of the patient involved.

REFERENCES

1. Physical activity and health: a report of the Surgeon General. McLean (VA): International Medical Publishing; 1996.
2. Haskell WL, Lee I, Pate RR, et al. Physical activity and public health: updated recommendation for adults from the American college of sports medicine and the American heart association. Circulation 2007;116:1081–93.
3. Nelson ME, Rejeski WJ, Blair SN, et al. Physical activity and public health in older adults: recommendation from the American College of Sports Medicine and the American Heart Association. Circulation 2007;116:1094–105.
4. Nelson ME, Rejeski WJ, Blair SN, et al. Physical activity and public health in older adults: recommendation from the American College of Sports Medicine and the American Heart Association. Med Sci Sports Exerc 2007;39:1435–45.
5. Zhang W, Doherty M. EULAR recommendations for knee and hip osteoarthritis: a critique of the methodology. Br J Sports Med 2006;40:664–9.
6. Alonso J, Ferrer M, Gandek B, et al. Health-related quality of life associated with chronic conditions in eight countries: results from the International Quality of Life Assessment (IQOLA) Project RID A-5514-2010. Quality of Life Research 2004;13:283–98.

7. Fautrel B, Hilliquin P, Rozenberg S, et al. Impact of osteoarthritis: results of a nationwide survey of 10,000 patients consulting for OA. Joint Bone Spine 2005;72: 235–40.
8. Kurtz S, Ong K, Lau E, et al. Projections of primary and revision hip and knee arthroplasty in the United States from 2005 to 2030. J Bone Joint Surg Am 2007;89: 780–5.
9. Otten R, van Roermund PM, Picavet HS. Trends in the number of knee and hip arthroplasties: considerably more knee and hip prostheses due to osteoarthritis in 2030. Ned Tijdschr Geneeskd 2010;154:A1534.
10. Schmalzried T, Shepherd E, Dorey F, et al. Wear is a function of use, not time. Clin Orthop 2000;381:36–46.
11. Schmalzried T, Huk O. Patient factors and wear in total hip arthroplasty. Clin Orthop 2004;418:94–7.
12. Muenger P, Roeder C, Ackermann-Liebrich U, et al. Patient-related risk factors leading to aseptic stem loosening in total hip arthroplasty: a case-control study of 5,035 patients. Acta Orthopaedica 2006;77:567–74.
13. Warburton D, Gledhill N, Quinney A. Musculoskeletal fitness and health. Can J Appl Physiol 2001;26:217–37.
14. Warburton D, Gledhill N, Quinney A. The effects of changes in musculoskeletal fitness on health. Can J Appl Physiol 2001;26:161–216.
15. Warburton D, Nicol C, Bredin S. Health benefits of physical activity: the evidence. Can Med Assoc J 2006;174:801–9.
16. Rowe J, Kahn R. Human aging: usual and successful. Science 1987;237:143–9.
17. Chang J, Morton S, Rubenstein L, et al. Interventions for the prevention of falls in older adults: systematic review and meta-analysis of randomised clinical trials. Br Med J 2004;328:680–3.
18. Gregg E, Pereira M, Caspersen C. Physical activity, falls, and fractures among older adults: a review of the epidemiologic evidence. J Am Geriatr Soc 2000;48:883–93.
19. Kannus P, Parkkari J, Koskinen S, et al. Fall-induced injuries and deaths among older adults. JAMA 1999;281:1895–9.
20. Dubs L, Gschwend N, Munzinger U. Sport after total hip-arthroplasty. Arch Orthop Trauma Surg 1983;101:161–9.
21. Widhalm R, Hofer G, Krugluger J, et al. Is the risk of sports injury or the risk of osteoporosis due to inactivity greater in total hip cases: conclusions regarding the durability of prosthesis anchorage. Z Orthop Ihre 1990;128:139–43.
22. Gschwend N, Frei T, Morscher E, et al. Alpine and cross-country skiing after total hip replacement: 2 cohorts of 50 patients each, one active, the other inactive in skiing, followed for 5–10 years. Acta Orthop Scand 2000;71:243–9.
23. Rosenbaum TG, Bloebaum RD, Ashrafi S, et al. Ambulatory activities maintain cortical bone after total hip arthroplasty. Clin Orthop 2006;450:129–37.
24. Kuster M. Exercise recommendations after total joint replacement: a review of the current literature and proposal of scientifically based guidelines. Sports Med 2002; 32:433–45.
25. Surin V, Sundholm K. Survival of patients and prostheses after total hip-arthroplasty. Clin Orthop 1983;177:148–53.
26. Woodruff M, Stone M. Comparison of weight changes after total hip or knee arthroplasty. J Arthroplasty 2001;16:22–4.
27. Heisel C, Silva M, Dela Rosa M, et al. The effects of lower-extremity total joint replacement for arthritis on obesity. Orthopedics 2005;28:157–9.
28. McClung C, Zahiri C, Higa J, et al. Relationship between body mass index and activity in hip or knee arthroplasty patients. J Orthop Res 2000;18:35–9.

29. Dorey F. Survivorship analysis of surgical treatment of the hip in young patients. Clin Orthop 2004;418:23–8.
30. Sallis J, Saelens B. Assessment of physical activity by self-report: status, limitations, and future directions. Res Q Exerc Sport 2000;71:409.
31. Harris W, Krushell R, Galante J. Results of cementless revisions of total hip arthroplasties using the Harris-Galante prosthesis. Clin Orthop 1988;235:120–6.
32. Insall J, Dorr L, Scott R, et al. Rationale of the Knee-Society Clinical Rating System. Clin Orthop 1989;248:13–4.
33. Murray DW, Fitzpatrick R, Rogers K, et al. The use of the Oxford hip and knee scores. J Bone Joint Surg B 2007;89B:1010–4.
34. Roos E, Roos H, Lohmander L, et al. Knee injury and osteoarthritis outcome score (KOOS): development of a self-administered outcome measure. J Orthop Sports Phys Ther 1998;28:88–96.
35. Klassbo M, Larsson E, Mannevik E. Hip disability and osteoarthritis outcome score: an extension of the Western Ontario and McMaster Universities Osteoarthritis Index. Scand J Rheumatol 2003;32:46–51.
36. Bellamy N, Buchanan W, Goldsmith C, et al. Validation-study of WOMAC: a health-status instrument for measuring clinically important patient relevant outcomes to antirheumatic drug-therapy in patients with osteo-arthritis of the hip or knee. J Rheumatol 1988;15:1833–40.
37. Ware J, Sherbourne C. The Mos 36-Item Short-Form Health Survey (Sf-36) .1. Conceptual-framework and item selection. Med Care 1992;30:473–83.
38. Wagenmakers R, Stevens M, van den Akker-Scheek I, et al. Predictive value of the Western Ontario and McMaster Universities Osteoarthritis Index for the amount of physical activity after total hip arthroplasty. Phys Ther 2008;88:211–8.
39. Morlock M, Schneider E, Bluhm A, et al. Duration and frequency of every day activities in total hip patients. J Biomech 2001;34:873–81.
40. Sallis JF, Owen N. Physical activity & behavioral medicine. Thousand Oaks (CA): Sage; 1999.
41. Amstutz H, Thomas B, Jinnah R, et al. Treatment of primary osteoarthritis of the hip: a comparison of total joint and surface replacement arthroplasty. J Bone Joint Surg A 1984;66A:228–41.
42. Grimby G. Physical-activity and muscle training in the elderly. Acta Med Scand 1986;711:233–7.
43. Craig C, Marshall A, Sjostrom M, et al. International physical activity questionnaire: 12-country reliability and validity. Med Sci Sports Exerc 2003;35:1381–95.
44. Wendel-Vos G, Schuit A, Saris W, et al. Reproducibility and relative validity of the Short Questionnaire to assess health-enhancing physical activity. J Clin Epidemiol 2003;56:1163–9.
45. Wagenmakers R, van den Akker-Scheek I, Groothoff JW, et al. Reliability and validity of the short questionnaire to assess health-enhancing physical activity (SQUASH) in patients after total hip arthroplasty. BMC Musculoskelet Disord 2008;9:141.
46. Esliger DW, Tremblay MS. Physical activity and inactivity profiling: the next generation. Appl Physiol Nutr Metab 2007;32:S195–207.
47. Hu FB. Sedentary lifestyle and risk of obesity and type 2 diabetes. Lipids 2003;38:103–8.
48. Veerman JL, Healy GN, Cobiac LJ, et al. Television viewing time and reduced life expectancy: a life table analysis. Br J Sports Med 2011. [Epub ahead of print].
49. Gardiner PA, Healy GN, Eakin EG, et al. Associations between television viewing time and overall sitting time with the metabolic syndrome in older men and women: the Australian Diabetes, Obesity and Lifestyle study. J Am Geriatr Soc 2011;59:788–96.

50. Wijndaele K, Healy GN, Dunstan DW, et al. Increased cardiometabolic risk is associated with increased TV viewing time. Med Sci Sports Exerc 2010;42:1511–8.

51. Winkler EA, Gardiner PA, Clark BK, et al. Identifying sedentary time using automated estimates of accelerometer wear time. Br J Sports Med 2012;46:436–42.

52. Wagenmakers R, Stevens M, Zijlstra W, et al. Habitual physical activity behavior of patients after primary total hip arthroplasty. Phys Ther 2008;88:1039–48.

53. Wagenmakers R, Stevens M, Groothoff JW, et al. Physical activity behavior of patients 1 year after primary total hip arthroplasty: a prospective multicenter cohort study. Phys Ther 2011;91:373–80.

54. Bauman S, Williams D, Petruccelli D, et al. Physical activity after total joint replacement: a cross-sectional survey. Clin J Sport Med 2007;17:104–8.

55. Beaule P, Dorey F, Hoke R, et al. The value of patient activity level in the outcome of total hip arthroplasty. J Arthroplasty 2006;21:547–52.

56. Sechriest VF 2nd, Kyle RF, Marek DJ, et al. Activity level in young patients with primary total hip arthroplasty: a 5-year minimum follow-up. J Arthroplasty 2007;22:39–47.

57. Chatterji U, Ashworth M, Lewis P, et al. Effect of total hip arthroplasty on recreational and sporting activity. ANZ J Surg 2004;74:446–9.

58. Nilsdotter AK, Toksvig-Larsen S, Roos EM. Knee arthroplasty: are patients' expectations fulfilled? Acta Orthopaedica 2009;80:55–61.

59. Dahm DL, Barnes SA, Harrington JR, et al. Patient-reported activity level after total knee arthroplasty. J Arthroplasty 2008;23:401–7.

60. Marker DR, Mont MA, Seyler TM, et al. Does functional improvement following TKA correlate to increased sports activity? Iowa Orthop J 2009;29:11–6.

61. Brandes M, Ringling M, Winter C, et al. Changes in physical activity and health-related quality of life during the first year after total knee arthroplasty. Arthritis Care Res 2011;63:328–34.

62. McGrory B, Stuart M, Sim F. Participation in sports after hip and knee arthroplasty - review of literature and survey of surgeon preferences. Mayo Clin Proc 1995;70: 342–8.

63. Swanson EA, Schmalzried TP, Dorey FJ. Activity recommendations after total hip and knee arthroplasty: a survey of the American Association for Hip and Knee Surgeons. J Arthroplasty 2009;24:120–6.

64. Klein GR, Levine BR, Hozack WJ, et al. Return to athletic activity after total hip arthroplasty: consensus guidelines based on a survey of the Hip Society and American Association of Hip and Knee Surgeons. J Arthroplasty 2007;22:171–5.

65. Healy W, Iorio R, Lemos M. Athletic activity after total knee arthroplasty. Clin Orthop 2000;380:65–71.

66. Healy W, Iorio R, Lemos M. Athletic activity after joint replacement. Am J Sports Med 2001;29:377–88.

67. Stevens M, Hagen H. Een Nieuwe Heup of Knie: Hoe Wordt u Lichamelijk En Sportief Weer Actief? Houten: Bohn Stafleu van Loghum; 2011.

68. Schmitt-Sody M, Pilger V, Gerdesmeyer L. Rehabilitation and sport following total hip replacement. Orthopade 2011;40:513–9.

Race/Ethnicity and Use of Elective Joint Replacement in the Management of End-Stage Knee/Hip Osteoarthritis
A Review of the Literature

Marissa A. Blum, MD, MS[a],*, Said A. Ibrahim, MD, MPH[b,c]

KEYWORDS

- Disparity • Joint arthroplasty • Osteoarthritis • Race/ethnicity

KEY POINTS

- Osteoarthritis is the most prevalent form of arthritis for which elective knee and hip joint replacement are effective treatment options in the management of end-stage knee/hip osteoarthritis; there are, however, marked racial disparities in the utilization of joint arthroplasty.
- Multiple studies have shown that insurance and access to care are not necessarily underlying causes for these disparities; other studies have shown that there are real and significant differences between racial/ethnic groups in preferences for and expectations of joint arthroplasty.
- Research has established there are racial differences in certain postoperative processes and outcomes. Reasons have not been elucidated, but highlight the need for more research to understand these differences and their causes, and then to design interventions to minimize these inequalities.

HEALTH IMPACT OF KNEE AND HIP OSTEOARTHRITIS

Osteoarthritis (OA) is the most common type of arthritis, causing pain, disability, and an overall diminished quality of life in patients.[1,2] The prevalence of OA varies depending on whether OA is defined clinically or radiographically. Radiographic

The authors have nothing to disclose.
[a] Division of Rheumatology, Temple University School of Medicine, 3322 North Broad Street, Suite 205, Philadelphia, PA 19140, USA; [b] Department of Medicine, Philadelphia VA Medical Center, 3900 Woodland Avenue, Philadelphia, PA 19104, USA; [c] Department of Medicine, The University of Pennsylvania School of Medicine, Blockley Hall, 12th Floor, Curie Boulevard, Philadelphia, PA, USA
* Corresponding author.
E-mail address: Marissa.blum@tuhs.temple.edu

definitions are further confounded by structural changes that may occur as patients age.[1] Symptomatic knee and hip OA as defined by symptoms and radiographic changes has been estimated to occur in 12% and 17% and up to 9% of adults over the age of 45, respectively.[3-5] Several studies have shown that African Americans have a higher burden of radiographic knee OA than their white counterparts,[3,6] and 1 study has shown equivalent rates of radiographic hip OA.[5] In a recent study evaluating patients with self-reported arthritis, African-American and Hispanic patients reported a lower prevalence of doctor-diagnosed arthritis, but a greater impact on activity level, work limitation, and severe joint pain.[7]

The burden of OA continues to grow. A recent study projected the prevalence of OA may increase to 25% of the adult population by 2030.[8] Another study estimated that the lifetime risk for patients is 50% by age 85 and most predicted by the presence of obesity.[9] The risk for developing OA is in part an age-dependent process, but has also been associated with trauma, genetics, obesity, and other lifestyle and occupational factors.[10]

TREATMENT OF LOWER EXTREMITY OA

Currently, there is no known cure for OA of the knee or hip. Pharmacologic therapy is limited to analgesics such as acetaminophen or anti-inflammatories; however, these drugs are not disease-modifying agents. Oral nutritional supplements such as glucosamine or chondroitin have not been shown to help the pain or progression of lower extremity OA.[11] Nonpharmacologic therapies such as exercise or physical therapy may be helpful for pain control and functioning, and intra-articular corticosteroid injections or viscosupplementation with hyaluronic acid derivatives may also help with short-term control of symptoms, but none of these modalities are curative.[12]

Today, the definitive treatment for lower extremity OA is total joint arthroplasty (TJA). Since both were first performed, total hip and knee replacement each have been demonstrated to improve pain, function, and quality of life in end-stage joint OA.[13-16] The success of TJA is reflected by the wide spread utilization of this treatment. In 2007, approximately 543,000 primary knee replacements and 230,000 primary hip replacements were performed in the United States alone.[17]

RACIAL DISPARITIES IN JOINT REPLACEMENT

Despite the huge burden of OA of the lower extremities and the proven effectiveness of knee and hip replacement in reducing symptoms and improving quality of life for OA patients, there are inequalities between African-American and white patients in the care of lower extremity OA. Disparities have been demonstrated at multiple levels in the care of these patients, including in the utilization of arthroplasty, postoperative care, and arthroplasty outcomes. The reasons are complex and not fully elucidated. The next several sections elaborate on these disparities and some of the reasons they might exist.

Joint Replacement Utilization

Many studies have documented the presence of racial/ethnic differences in the utilization of knee or hip joint replacement over the past 15 to 20 years, with African-American patients consistently underutilizing joint replacement surgery for OA of the lower extremity compared with their white counterparts.[18-27] Most of these studies have utilized Medicare data where patients are generally age 65 or older, and access to the procedure based on insurance status is not a significant issue.[18,19,22]

Disparities have also been demonstrated in samples other than the Medicare population after controlling for insurance or other financial access variables.[20,21,28] One study using the Longitudinal Health and Retirement Survey showed that African Americans were less likely to undergo hip or knee replacement if they were older ($\geq$65 years), but not younger after adjusting for income, wealth, education, and insurance.[28] Data from the National Inpatient Survey showed these disparities exist regardless of age after controlling for income as a marker of socioeconomic status.[27]

Inequalities in rates of use of hip replacement have also been demonstrated in other racial/ethnic groups.[27] Hoaglund and colleagues[21] showed that hip replacement rates were lower for Asians, Hispanics, and African Americans compared with Caucasian patients in a study based on hospital data from San Francisco. In 2 separate studies using hospital records data from Texas and Medicare data, Escalante and associates[23,24] showed that Hispanics, compared with other racial/ethnic groups, were less likely to undergo hip replacement. Skinner and associates[29] showed a lower odds of undergoing knee replacement for Asian, Hispanic, and African-American men and Asian women when compared with white men.

The Racial Gap Is Growing

Although these studies have demonstrated that disparities exist, some more recent studies have shown that, despite this knowledge and widespread awareness and initiative to reduce disparities,[30] the gap has grown. In a study of hospital discharge data from Pennsylvania and New York from 1997 to 2001, Basu and colleagues[31] evaluated all patients older than age 65 who had insurance other than Medicare fee for service, and found that disparities in the utilization of hip/joint replacement among elderly patients of other races relative to whites worsen over time in this population. African Americans compared with white patients were 24% less likely to receive a joint replacement in 1997 and 46% less likely in 2001.[31] Most recently, however, the US Centers for Disease Control and Prevention analyzed national and state total knee replacement Medicare data from 2000 to 2006. They found that the TKA rate in 2000 was 37% lower for African Americans than whites, which compares with 2006, where the disparity grew to 39%[32] (**Fig. 1**).

REASONS FOR RACIAL/ETHNIC DISPARITIES IN JOINT REPLACEMENT UTILIZATION

The reasons for racial/ethnic disparities in utilization of joint arthroplasty as an effective option for hip and knee OA remain unknown, but include factors at the patient, provider, and health system levels. Additionally, there are a number of potentially interrelated factors affecting utilization of health services after patients have entered the health system. Some of these factors include patient preferences for and expectations of procedures.

Patient Preferences

Patient preferences have been shown to contribute to racial/ethnic differences in utilization of other medical procedures.[33,34] In a study of male Veterans Affairs' (VA) patients with OA, Ibrahim and colleagues[35] evaluated racial differences in perception of the efficacy of treatments and self-care for arthritis. They found that African Americans, compared with white patients, were more likely to rely on self-care modalities for treatment of OA, and perceived less invasive treatments such as physical therapy and complementary therapies as more effective for OA treatment than white patients.[35] Additionally, African-American patients perceived knee or hip replacement as less effective for OA than white patients.[35] In another related study

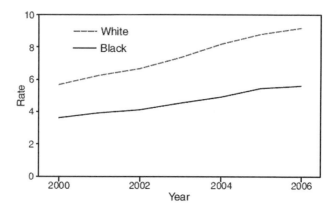

* Per 1,000 population. Age-adjusted to the United States 2000 projected population.
† Defined as *International Classification of Diseases, Ninth Revision, Clinical Modification* code 81.54 (total knee replacement) on hospital claims records from acute care, short-term hospitals.
§ U.S. residents in the 50 states or District of Columbia who were aged ≥65 years, entitled for Medicare Part A, and not members of managed care organizations.

Fig. 1. Age-adjusted rates* of total knee replacement† among Medicare enrollees,§ by white or black race in the United States, 2000 to 2006. (*From* Centers for Disease Control and Prevention. Racial disparities in total knee replacement among Medicare enrollees—United States, 2000–2006. MMWR 2009;58:133–8.)

using the "willingness to pay" concept, Ibrahim and colleagues[36] investigated whether African Americans differed from white patients in willingness to consider joint replacement if the procedure was indicated. "Willingness" is best viewed as a sum of clinical, social, and personal factors. In this study, they found that African-American patients were less willing to consider joint replacement surgery; however, differences in expectations of surgery explained some of this.[36] In another willingness to pay study based in Texas, Byrne and colleagues[37] found that willingness to pay for treatment of OA varied significantly between racial groups, suggesting that racial/ethnic differences in the value patients place on these health conditions contributes to utilization of health services to treat OA. Another study from the same group showed that patient preferences were significantly different between racial groups, and remained significant factors for considering joint replacement after controlling for other demographic factors.[38] Most recently, Hausmann and colleagues also[39] found that patient preference for joint replacement mediated the difference in total joint replacement recommendations by orthopedic physicians and subsequent utilization of the procedure.

Given that joint arthroplasty is considered an elective procedure, it makes sense that patient preference has an important role here. What affects patient preferences for OA care is shaped largely by patients' local environment, including personal experiences, expectations, fears, social interactions, explanations of illness, trust, skepticism, and financial burden[40–42] (**Fig. 2**).

Patient Expectations

Patient expectations of treatment outcomes may mediate preferences. Many studies have evaluated racial differences in expectations regarding joint arthroplasty to gain

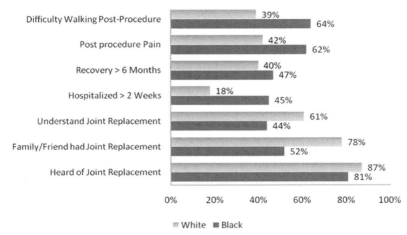

Fig. 2. Differences in expectations and knowledge of joint replacement between African-American and white patients with OA. (Reprinted with permission from Ibrahim SA, Siminoff LA, Burant CJ, et al. Understanding ethnic differences in the utilization of joint replacement for osteoarthritis: the role of patient-level factors. Med Care 2002;40(Suppl 1):I44–51.)

an understanding of how this affects utilization of the procedure. Expectations regarding improvement of knee pain and arthroplasty were evaluated by Figaro and colleagues.[43] In a cross-sectional survey of African-American patients with knee OA, only 36% believed that total knee replacement was likely to improve knee pain and 45% thought the procedure would improve walking.[43] A prior qualitative study by the same author also discovered African-American patients have low expectations of total knee replacement.[44] African-American patients perceived it as either ineffective therapy for themselves or had seen it as ineffective for others.[44] In another cross-sectional study of male VA patients with OA, African-American patients were less familiar with joint arthroplasty as a treatment for OA and had lower expectations for successful postoperative course with concerns about a prolonged hospitalization, and moderate to severe pain and difficulty walking after joint replacement compared with white patients.[42] Even after controlling for other potential confounders such as health literacy, social support, educational attainment, and trust in physicians, Groeneveld and colleagues[45] found that African-American patients still had lower expectations for outcomes after joint replacement surgery (**Fig. 3**).

Other Patient Factors

Other factors potentially affecting utilization of joint arthroplasty may not directly have to do with expectations or preferences, but instead relate to patient traits. One important question investigated in the literature is this: Are there racial/ethnic differences in how patients cope with OA pain? Ang and colleagues[46] found that African Americans and white patients with OA do not seem to have differences in the amount of symptoms by OA radiographic class, suggesting that there are no racial differences in the perception of symptoms. However, in a separate study Ibrahim and colleagues[47] found that African-American patients with OA describe the quality of OA pain differently from white patients. Lavernia and associates[48] evaluated pain-related anxiety, including fear about consequences of pain, in patients with lower extremity OA and found racial differences as well, with African-American patients having higher

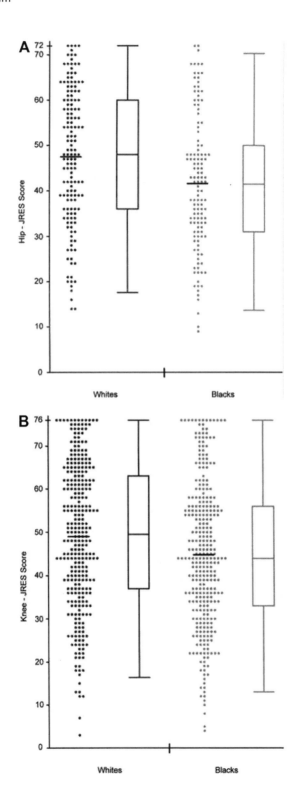

levels of both anxiety and fear compared with white patients.[48] In another study from Canada, non-European patients (Asian and black) with lower extremity OA had greater perception of surgical risk compared with those of European descent.[49]

In another study, Jones and colleagues[50] evaluated racial differences in coping with pain and self-efficacy for OA patients. The authors found that African Americans relied more on prayer and hope as a strategy to manage OA related pain. Ang and co-workers[51] also studied the role of prayer/religiosity on the management of OA and found African Americans were more likely to consider prayer as helpful to their OA management.

RACIAL/ETHNIC DISPARITIES IN JOINT REPLACEMENT OUTCOMES

Less well-studied but important to define are any racial/ethnic variations in outcomes postarthroplasty. Most randomized, prospective trials do not report race as a covariate when analyzing data[52,53]; however, given that patient preferences, expectations, and other patient-level factors differ between races and affect arthroplasty utilization, evaluating arthroplasty outcomes by race are valid as well.

Nwachukwu and colleagues[54] recently published a comprehensive review on complications for patients after joint arthroplasty by race. There were only a handful of studies evaluating mortality and although there seemed to be an increased risk for African-American patients after hip and knee replacement in 2 studies by Mahomed and colleagues,[55,56] 2 separate studies did not find any difference between races for hip or knee replacement mortality rates.[57,58] Infection risk after hip replacement was conflicted[55,59]; however, after knee replacement, 3 studies showed an increased risk of postoperative infection among nonwhite patients.[56,58,59] Several studies found that after both hip and knee replacement, nonwhite patients had greater duration of stay.[60–62]

In studies of noninfectious complications, such as pulmonary embolus or readmission post hip replacement, 2 studies found no significant difference in racial groups.[55,59] The data show different results for knee replacement noninfectious complications. Two studies found that nonwhite patients were more likely to have complications within 30 days of the procedure.[59,61] Another study found an increased risk of pulmonary embolism for African-American compared with white patients, but not for Hispanic patients after knee replacement,[58] and another study found an increased risk of readmission to acute care facility within 90 days postarthroplasty.[56] Recently, we showed that the 1- and 5-year knee replacement revision risk is greater for African-American compared with white patients (Blum et al, unpublished data, 2012), lending support to a prior study demonstrating higher revision risk for knee replacement for African-American compared with white patients.[63]

Compared with complication outcomes, functional outcomes have been even less well studied between African-American and white patients; however, 2 studies by Lavernia and associates[48] offer some insight. In 1 prospective cohort study of patients with end-stage OA who underwent hip or knee replacement, African-American patients had worse functional scores as measured by the SF-36 both pre-

---

Fig. 3. Racial/ethnic differences in Joint Replacement Expectations Score (JRES) for (A) hip and (B) knee replacement. (Reprinted with permission from Groeneveld PW, Kwoh CK, Mor MK, et al. Racial differences in expectations of joint replacement surgery outcomes. Arthritis Rheum 2008;59:730–7.)

and postoperatively compared with white patients.[48] In a retrospective review, the authors found that both pre- and postarthroplasty, nonwhite patients had worse functional scores, Western Ontario and McMaster Universities Osteoarthritis Index scores, and quality-of-life scores.[64]

Racial/Ethnic Disparities in Processes of Care

Although most effort has been spent evaluating inequalities of utilization of TJA and complications postarthroplasty, several other areas of disparity research are worthwhile to mention because they provide foci for future interventions, either as quality initiatives or as policy or public health changes to eliminate disparities of care and improve outcomes.

Differences in hospital quality have been evaluated for sources of disparity by 2 authors. SooHoo and colleagues[65] analyzed hospital discharge data from California and found that racial/ethnic minority patients, including African-American, Hispanic and Asian/Pacific Islander, compared with white patients were more likely to undergo joint replacement at a low-volume hospital as opposed to a high-volume hospital. In another study of Medicare patients, Cai and colleagues[66] found that African-American patients undergoing a knee replacement were significantly more likely to be admitted to hospitals with higher risk adjusted postoperative rates of complications or mortality. Both studies suggest racial/ethnic minorities have their joint arthroplasties at hospitals with poorer quality of care.

Postarthroplasty care has not been well studied for disparities, but 1 study from 2003 showed no major differences between white and African-American patients for discharge to inpatient rehabilitation.[67] A more recent study that evaluated postarthroplasty rehabilitation by analyzing hospital discharge data from 4 states, found that racial minorities receive less intensive postarthroplasty care.[68] The effects were modified slightly by insurance and state.[68]

In another study of VA patients, Lopez and associates[69] evaluated how difficult it is for patients with lower extremity OA to obtain specialty OA services. They found that African Americans perceived a less difficult time in attaining medical care compared with white patients, which may reflect physical access to the VA facility, rather than access to care.

Finally, the quality of communication between OA patients and their providers has also been studied. Qualitative work by Levinson and co-workers[70] analyzing taped patient encounters between orthopedic providers and their patients found that African-American patients had worse scores for communication with the surgeon and overall satisfaction of the visit compared with white patients, but similar scores for informed decision making. In another study among VA patients, Hausmann and colleagues[71] found that there were few racial differences in patient–surgeon communications in the orthopedic setting.

SUMMARY

Although much research has documented disparities exist for utilization of TJA, additional studies have shown that we have not narrowed the gap. Because multiple studies have shown that insurance and access to care are not necessarily underlying causes for these disparities, other studies have shown that there are real and significant differences between racial/ethnic groups in preferences for and expectations of joint arthroplasty. Additional research has established there are racial differences in certain postoperative processes and outcomes. Reasons have not been elucidated, but highlight the need for more research to understand these differences, their causes, and then to design interventions to minimize these inequalities.

REFERENCES

1. Lawrence RC, Felson DT, Helmick CG, et al. Estimates of the prevalence of arthritis and other rheumatic conditions in the United States. Arthritis Rheum 2008;58:26–35.
2. Dominick KL, Ahern FM, Gold CH, et al. Health-related quality of life among older adults with arthritis. Health Qual Life Outcomes 2004;2:5.
3. Dillon CF, Rasch EK, Gu Q, et al. Prevalence of knee osteoarthritis in the United States: arthritis data from the Third National Health and Nutrition Examination Survey 1991-94. J Rheumatol 2006;33:2271–9.
4. Jordan JM, Helmick CG, Renner JB, et al. Prevalence of knee symptoms and radiographic and symptomatic knee osteoarthritis in African Americans and Caucasians: the Johnston County Osteoarthritis Project. J Rheumatol 2007;34:172–80.
5. Helmick CG, Renner JB, Luta G, et al. Prevalence of hip pain, radiographic hip osteoarthritis (OA), severe radiographic hip OA, and symptomatic hip OA: the Johnson County Osteoarthritis Project [Abstract]. Arthritis Rheum 2003;48(Suppl):S212.
6. Sowers M, Lachance L, Hochberg M, et al. Radiographically defined osteoarthritis of the hand and knee in young and middle-aged African American and Caucasian women. Osteoarthritis Cartilage 2000;8:69–77.
7. Bolen J, Schieb L, Hootman JM, et al. Differences in the prevalence and severity of arthritis among racial/ethnic groups in the United States, National Health Interview Survey, 2002, 2003, and 2006. Prev Chronic Dis 2010;7:A64.
8. Hootman JM, Helmick CG. Projections of US prevalence of arthritis and associated activity limitations. Arthritis Rheum 2006;54:226–9.
9. Murphy L, Schwartz TA, Helmick CG, et al. Lifetime risk of symptomatic knee osteoarthritis. Arthritis Rheum 2008;59:1207–13.
10. Hochberg MC, Altman RD, Brandt KD, et al. Guidelines for the medical management of osteoarthritis. Part I. Osteoarthritis of the hip. American College of Rheumatology. Arthritis Rheum 1995;38:1535–40.
11. Wandel S, Juni P, Tendal B, et al. Effects of glucosamine, chondroitin, or placebo in patients with osteoarthritis of hip or knee: network meta-analysis. bmj 2010;341:c4675.
12. Zhang W, Nuki G, Moskowitz RW, et al. OARSI recommendations for the management of hip and knee osteoarthritis: part III: changes in evidence following systematic cumulative update of research published through January 2009. Osteoarthritis Cartilage 2010;18:476–99.
13. Hawker G, Wright J, Coyte P, et al. Health-related quality of life after knee replacement. Results of the knee replacement patient outcomes research study team. J of Bone Joint Surg 1998;80:163–73.
14. Singh J, Sloan JA, Johanson NA. Challenges with health-related quality of life assessment in arthroplasty patients: problems and solutions. J Am Acad Orthop Surg 2010;18:72–82.
15. Ethgen O, Bruyere O, Richy F, et al. Health-related quality of life in total hip and total knee arthroplasty. A qualitative and systematic review of the literature. J Bone Joint Surg Am 2004;86-A:963-74.
16. Hamel MB, Toth M, Legedza A, et al. Joint replacement surgery in elderly patients with severe osteoarthritis of the hip or knee: decision making, postoperative recovery, and clinical outcomes. Arch Intern Med 2008;168:1430–40.
17. Hall MJ, DeFrances CJ, Williams SN, et al. National Hospital Discharge Survey: 2007 summary. Natl Health Stat Report 2010;29:1.

18. Escarce JJ, Epstein KR, Colby DC, et al. Racial differences in the elderly's use of medical procedures and diagnostic tests. Am J Public Health 1993;83:948–54.

19. Baron JA, Barrett J, Katz JN, et al. Total hip arthroplasty: use and select complications in the US Medicare population. Am J Public Health 1996;86:70–2.

20. Sharkness CM, Hamburger S, Moore RM Jr, et al. Prevalence of artificial hip implants and use of health services by recipients. Public Health Rep 1993;108:70–5.

21. Hoaglund FT, Oishi CS, Gialamas GG. Extreme variations in racial rates of total hip arthroplasty for primary coxarthrosis: a population-based study in San Francisco. Ann Rheum Dis 1995;54:107–10.

22. Katz BP, Freund DA, Heck DA, et al. Demographic variation in the rate of knee replacement: a multi-year analysis. Health Serv Res 1996;31:125–40.

23. Escalante A, Espinosa-Morales R, del Rincon I, et al. Recipients of hip replacement for arthritis are less likely to be Hispanic, independent of access to health care and socioeconomic status. Arthritis Rheum 2000;43:390–9.

24. Escalante A, Barrett J, del Rincon I, et al. Disparity in total hip replacement affecting Hispanic Medicare beneficiaries. Med Care 2002;40:451–60.

25. Steel N, Clark A, Lang IA, et al. Racial disparities in receipt of hip and knee joint replacements are not explained by need: the Health and Retirement Study 1998–2004. J Gerontol A Biol Sci Med Sci 2008;63:629–34.

26. Skinner J, Weinstein JN, Sporer SM, et al. Racial, ethnic, and geographic disparities in rates of knee arthroplasty among Medicare patients. N Engl J Med 2003;349:1350–9.

27. Bang H, Chiu YL, Memtsoudis SG, et al. Total hip and total knee arthroplasties: trends and disparities revisited. Am J Orthop (Belle Mead NJ) 2010;39:E95–102.

28. Dunlop DD, Manheim LM, Song J, et al. Age and racial/ethnic disparities in arthritis-related hip and knee surgeries. Med Care 2008;46:200–8.

29. Skinner J, Zhou W, Weinstein J. The influence of income and race on total knee arthroplasty in the United States. J Bone Joint Surg Am 2006;88:2159–66.

30. US Department of Health and Human Services. Healthy people 2010, 2nd edition, with understanding and improving health and objectives for improving health. Washington, DC: US Government Printing Office.

31. Basu J, Mobley LR. Trends in racial disparities among the elderly for selected procedures. Med Care Res Rev 2008;65:617–37.

32. US Centers for Disease Control and Prevention (CDC). Racial disparities in total knee replacement among Medicare enrollees: United States, 2000–2006. MMWR 2009;58:133–8.

33. Ayanian JZ, Cleary PD, Weissman JS, et al. The effect of patients' preferences on racial differences in access to renal transplantation. N Engl J Med 1999;341:1661–9.

34. Ashton CM, Haidet P, Paterniti DA, et al. Racial and ethnic disparities in the use of health services: bias, preferences, or poor communication? J Gen Intern Med 2003;18:146–52.

35. Ibrahim SA, Siminoff LA, Burant CJ, et al. Variation in perceptions of treatment and self-care practices in elderly with osteoarthritis: a comparison between African American and white patients. Arthritis Rheum 2001;45:340–5.

36. Ibrahim SA, Siminoff LA, Burant CJ, et al. Differences in expectations of outcome mediate African American/white patient differences in "willingness" to consider joint replacement. Arthritis Rheum 2002;46:2429–35.

37. Byrne MM, O'Malley KJ, Suarez-Almazor ME. Ethnic differences in health preferences: analysis using willingness-to-pay. J Rheumatol 2004;31:1811–8.

38. Suarez-Almazor ME, Souchek J, Kelly PA, et al. Ethnic variation in knee replacement: patient preferences or uninformed disparity? Arch Intern Med 2005;165:1117–24.

39. Hausmann LR, Mor M, Hanusa BH, et al. The effect of patient race on total joint replacement recommendations and utilization in the orthopedic setting. J Gen Intern Med 2010;25:982–8.

40. Kroll TL, Richardson M, Sharf BF, et al. "Keep on truckin'" or "It's got you in this little vacuum": race-based perceptions in decision-making for total knee arthroplasty. J Rheumatol 2007;34:1069–75.

41. Suarez-Almazor ME, Richardson M, Kroll TL, et al. A qualitative analysis of decision-making for total knee replacement in patients with osteoarthritis. J Clin Rheumatol 2010;16:158–63.

42. Ibrahim SA, Siminoff LA, Burant CJ, et al. Understanding ethnic differences in the utilization of joint replacement for osteoarthritis: the role of patient-level factors. Med Care 2002;40(Suppl 1):I44–51.

43. Figaro MK, Williams-Russo P, Allegrante JP. Expectation and outlook: the impact of patient preference on arthritis care among African Americans. J Ambul Care Manage 2005;28:41–8.

44. Figaro MK, Russo PW, Allegrante JP. Preferences for arthritis care among urban African Americans: "I don't want to be cut". Health Psychol 2004;23:324–9.

45. Groeneveld PW, Kwoh CK, Mor MK, et al. Racial differences in expectations of joint replacement surgery outcomes. Arthritis Rheum 2008;59:730–7.

46. Ang DC, Ibrahim SA, Burant CJ, et al. Is there a difference in the perception of symptoms between African Americans and whites with osteoarthritis? J Rheumatol 2003;30:1305–10.

47. Ibrahim SA, Burant CJ, Mercer MB, et al. Older patients' perceptions of quality of chronic knee or hip pain: differences by ethnicity and relationship to clinical variables. J Gerontol A Biol Sci Med Sci 2003;58:M472–7.

48. Lavernia CJ, Alcerro JC, Rossi MD. Fear in arthroplasty surgery: the role of race. Clin Orthop Relat Res 2010;468:547–54.

49. Gandhi R, Razak F, Davey JR, et al. Ethnicity and patient's perception of risk in joint replacement surgery. J Rheumatol 2008;35:1664–7.

50. Jones AC, Kwoh CK, Groeneveld PW, et al. Investigating racial differences in coping with chronic osteoarthritis pain. J Cross Cult Gerontol 2008;23:339–47.

51. Ang DC, Ibrahim SA, Burant CJ, et al. Ethnic differences in the perception of prayer and consideration of joint arthroplasty. Med Care 2002;40:471–6.

52. Barton TM, Gleeson R, Topliss C, et al. A comparison of the long gamma nail with the sliding hip screw for the treatment of AO/OTA 31-A2 fractures of the proximal part of the femur: a prospective randomized trial. J Bone Joint Surg Am 2010;92:792–8.

53. Demey G, Servien E, Pinaroli A, et al. The influence of femoral cementing on perioperative blood loss in total knee arthroplasty: a prospective randomized study. J Bone Joint Surg Am 2010;92:536–41.

54. Nwachukwu BU, Kenny AD, Losina E, et al. Complications for racial and ethnic minority groups after total hip and knee replacement: a review of the literature. J Bone Joint Surg Am 2010;92:338–45.

55. Mahomed NN, Barrett JA, Katz JN, et al. Rates and outcomes of primary and revision total hip replacement in the United States Medicare population. J Bone Joint Surg Am 2003;85-A:27-32.

56. Mahomed NN, Barrett J, Katz JN, et al. Epidemiology of total knee replacement in the United States Medicare population. J Bone Joint Surg Am 2005;87:1222–8.

57. Whittle J, Steinberg EP, Anderson GF, et al. Mortality after elective total hip arthroplasty in elderly Americans. Age, gender, and indication for surgery predict survival. Clin Orthop Relat Res 1993;295:119–26.

58. SooHoo NF, Lieberman JR, Ko CY, et al. Factors predicting complication rates following total knee replacement. J Bone Joint Surg Am 2006;88:480–5.
59. Ibrahim SA, Stone RA, Han X, et al. Racial/ethnic differences in surgical outcomes in veterans following knee or hip arthroplasty. Arthritis Rheum 2005;52:3143–51.
60. White RH, McCurdy SA, Marder RA. Early morbidity after total hip replacement: rheumatoid arthritis versus osteoarthritis. J Gen Intern Med 1990;5:304–9.
61. Weaver F, Hynes D, Hopkinson W, et al. Preoperative risks and outcomes of hip and knee arthroplasty in the Veterans Health Administration. J Arthroplasty 2003;18:693–708.
62. Collins TC, Daley J, Henderson WH, et al. Risk factors for prolonged length of stay after major elective surgery. Ann Surg 1999;230:251–9.
63. Ong KL, Lau E, Suggs J, et al. Risk of subsequent revision after primary and revision total joint arthroplasty. Clin Orthop Relat Res 2010;468:3070–6.
64. Lavernia CJ, Alcerro JC, Contreras JS, et al. Ethnic and racial factors influencing well-being, perceived pain, and physical function after primary total joint arthroplasty. Clin Orthop Relat Res 2011;469:1838–45.
65. SooHoo NF, Zingmond DS, Ko CY. Disparities in the utilization of high-volume hospitals for total knee replacement. J Natl Med Assoc 2008;100:559–64.
66. Cai X, Cram P, Vaughan-Sarrazin M. Are African American patients more likely to receive a total knee arthroplasty in a low-quality hospital? Clin Orthop Relat Res 2012;470:1185–93.
67. Ottenbacher KJ, Smith PM, Illig SB, et al. Disparity in health services and outcomes for persons with hip fracture and lower extremity joint replacement. Med Care 2003;41:232–41.
68. Freburger JK, Holmes GM, Ku LJ, et al. Disparities in post-acute rehabilitation care for joint replacement. Arthritis Care Res (Hoboken) 2011;63:1020–30.
69. Lopez JP, Burant CJ, Siminoff LA, et al. Patient perceptions of access to care and referrals to specialists: a comparison of African-American and white older patients with knee and hip osteoarthritis. J Natl Med Assoc 2005;97:667–73.
70. Levinson W, Hudak PL, Feldman JJ, et al. "It's not what you say . . .": racial disparities in communication between orthopedic surgeons and patients. Med Care 2008;46:410–6.
71. Hausmann LR, Hanusa BH, Kresevic DM, et al. Orthopedic communication about osteoarthritis treatment: does patient race matter? Arthritis Care Res (Hoboken) 2011;63:635–42.

Index

Note: Page numbers of article titles are in **boldface** type.

A

Accelerometry, to assess physical activity after total hip/knee arthroplasty, 513
Acetaminophen, for preoperative pain management, in total joint replacement, 461
Age, patient, and satisfaction with total hip arthroplasty, 357
    and satisfaction with total knee arthroplasty, 353
Analgesia, preemptive, for pain management, in total joint replacement, 464, 465
Anesthesia, operative, for pain management, in total joint replacement, 465–466
Arthroplasty, total. See *Total hip arthroplasty; Total knee arthroplasty.*

C

Corticosteroid injections, intraarticular, for preoperative pain management, in total
    joint replacement, 463

D

15D assessment, 421
Delirium, postoperative, following total joint replacement, 478

E

Elderly, cardiovascular complications in, following total joint replacement, 481
    complications and special considerations in, following total joint replacement,
       473–474
    minimally invasive total hip and knee arthroplasty in, implications for, **447–458**
    neurovascular injury in, following total joint replacement, 481–482
    periprosthetic fracture in, following total joint replacement, 478–479
    postoperative delirium in, following total joint replacement, 478
EQ-5D utility measure, 415–421
Expectations, of patient, and satisfaction with total knee arthroplasty, 353–354,
    357–358

F

Fracture, periprosthetic, following total joint replacement, 478–479

I

Infection, deep, in total knee and hip arthroplasty, 440–442, 443
    periprosthetic joint, following total joint replacement, 474–477
Injections, intraoperative, for pain management, in total joint replacement, 466

J

Joint fluid therapy, for preoperative pain management, in total joint replacement, 463–464

Clin Geriatr Med 28 (2012) 533–538
http://dx.doi.org/10.1016/S0749-0690(12)00063-8
0749-0690/12/$ – see front matter © 2012 Elsevier Inc. All rights reserved.

geriatric.theclinics.com

V

W